Amos M. Yinnon

Daring to Change: Exploring Spiritual Dimensions of Modern Medicine

Amos M. Yinnon

Daring to Change: Exploring Spiritual Dimensions of Modern Medicine

LAP LAMBERT Academic Publishing

Impressum / Imprint
Bibliografische Information der Deutschen Nationalbibliothek: Die Deutsche Nationalbibliothek verzeichnet diese Publikation in der Deutschen Nationalbibliografie; detaillierte bibliografische Daten sind im Internet über http://dnb.d-nb.de abrufbar.
Alle in diesem Buch genannten Marken und Produktnamen unterliegen warenzeichen-, marken- oder patentrechtlichem Schutz bzw. sind Warenzeichen oder eingetragene Warenzeichen der jeweiligen Inhaber. Die Wiedergabe von Marken, Produktnamen, Gebrauchsnamen, Handelsnamen, Warenbezeichnungen u.s.w. in diesem Werk berechtigt auch ohne besondere Kennzeichnung nicht zu der Annahme, dass solche Namen im Sinne der Warenzeichen- und Markenschutzgesetzgebung als frei zu betrachten wären und daher von jedermann benutzt werden dürften.

Bibliographic information published by the Deutsche Nationalbibliothek: The Deutsche Nationalbibliothek lists this publication in the Deutsche Nationalbibliografie; detailed bibliographic data are available in the Internet at http://dnb.d-nb.de.
Any brand names and product names mentioned in this book are subject to trademark, brand or patent protection and are trademarks or registered trademarks of their respective holders. The use of brand names, product names, common names, trade names, product descriptions etc. even without a particular marking in this work is in no way to be construed to mean that such names may be regarded as unrestricted in respect of trademark and brand protection legislation and could thus be used by anyone.

Coverbild / Cover image: www.ingimage.com

Verlag / Publisher:
LAP LAMBERT Academic Publishing
ist ein Imprint der / is a trademark of
OmniScriptum GmbH & Co. KG
Heinrich-Böcking-Str. 6-8, 66121 Saarbrücken, Deutschland / Germany
Email: info@lap-publishing.com

Herstellung: siehe letzte Seite /
Printed at: see last page
ISBN: 978-3-659-59258-4

Copyright © 2014 OmniScriptum GmbH & Co. KG
Alle Rechte vorbehalten. / All rights reserved. Saarbrücken 2014

Dedication

This book is dedicated to my parents, Leo and Eva van Praagh. Their sensitive consideration of other people's feelings, enthusiastic support for diligent study and passionate love of Israel put me on the path to becoming a physician in my native country. This book is also dedicated to my wife, Tamar A. Yinnon. She has been and continues to be my truest companion and her unwavering aspiration to attain the highest and most exalted values has served simultaneously as a source of modesty and inspiration. I owe her my deepest gratitude for our family and my personal and professional development. I also wish to pay tribute to Shaare Zedek Medical Center, Jerusalem: its combination of professionalism and adherence to the Halachah provides for a tradition of first-class patient care. This special hospital offers expert professional education of young physicians and simultaneously fosters personal development – as well as incubation of ideas such as expressed in this book. Foremost, I profoundly thank H.K.B.H, whose involvement in the inception and execution of this book can be traced in all pages.

Contents

Dedication		1
Contents		3
Disclosure		5
Introduction		7
Chapter 1	Symptoms as symbols: The woman with the broken arm	11
Chapter 2	Making sense of suffering: The baby with end stage renal disease	14
Chapter 3	Futile medicine? The elderly, dement patient on the respirator	17
Chapter 4	A hole in his heart	21
Chapter 5	More futile medicine? Reading between the lines	30
Chapter 6	Perforated bowel: The unexpected benefit of a second opinion	36
Chapter 7	CMV in pregnancy: Counseling with wisdom in the face of uncertainty	41
Chapter 8	Sexually transmitted infection: Fertile ground for thoughtful talk	49
Chapter 9	Fever of unknown origin	59
Chapter 10	Leprosy: drug toxicity only?	73
Chapter 11	Second generation syndrome	92
Chapter 12	Chronic fatigue syndrome: A case for complimentary medicine	101
Chapter 13	Chronic urinary tract infection: What if ovaries could speak?	109
Chapter 14	Peyronie's disease: Transforming weakness to strength	120
Chapter 15	A case of marital conflict and distress	138
Chapter 16	Suicide: A story of jealousy and ambition	149
Epilogue		168
Alphabetical list of Hebrew words and their meaning		171
Biography and references		172

Disclosure

Scientific journals usually require of the authors of publications to disclose conflict of interest. Usually, this indicates a conflict of financial interest. However, there are many more considerations that readers may and would like to know about when reading papers and quite likely a book as this. I therefore wish to disclose the following:

I was born in Israel and studied medicine (1972-1978) at the Hebrew University-Hadassah Medical School, Jerusalem, Israel's oldest medical school, after which I was drafted and spent several years as an army physician (1980-1984). I subsequently specialized in internal medicine (1984-1988) in Shaare Zedek Medical Center, Jerusalem and then sub-specialized in infectious diseases, first at the Department of Clinical Microbiology and Infectious Diseases at the Hadassah Medical Center, Jerusalem (1989-1990) and subsequently at the University of Rochester Medical Center, Rochester, NY (1990-1992). After returning to Israel I joined the infectious disease unit at Shaare Zedek Medical Center and served as its head for fourteen years (1994-2006), combining clinical care, teaching and research. Hospital epidemiology and infection control as well as appropriate antibiotic use were my prime clinical and research interests. In 2006 I was appointed chairman of the division of internal medicine, a position that entails patient care, administrative duties, running of the academic program, fostering of professional development of its attending physicians and residents, teaching and research. Internal medicine has been passing through a significant transitional period for the last two-three decades. These changes impact on my daily life as physician, teacher and health administrator and of necessity question my thinking regarding many health related issues.

Shaare Zedek Medical Center is a special hospital. Established in 1902, it combines professionalism with humanistic values, most likely because the hospital is run according to the Halachah, the Jewish code of conduct. Already as a medical student I was attracted to this special blend of professionalism and humanistic/religious atmosphere values, although I was not particularly religious at the time. The patient and his requirements are put squarely at the core of the hospital's interest: their physical and biomedical needs, but also their psychological, social and spiritual needs. Although no place is perfect and hospitals are definitely not, patients, their families and the staff are in general quite satisfied.

My wife and I married in 1975 and are members of Kibbutz Kalia, a communal settlement at the northern tip of the Dead Sea. Next to Kalia is the site where the Dead Sea Scrolls were found, remnants of parchments with biblical text buried in pottery in the year 70 AD. That year the Romans destroyed the community of scribes living at the site, as well as the second Temple in Jerusalem. The scrolls were discovered in 1947: because of the area's hot and dry climate, many pieces of parchment remained intact after nineteen centuries. These finds are considered as belonging to the greatest archeological discoveries of modern times.

We have one son and one daughter, both married and parents of children themselves. Over time we have become religiously observant, both parents and children. Although religious Judaism contains various sectors, include the Haredy and Hassidic ultra-orthodox denominations and modern national-orthodox sector, we identify with various aspects of all sectors in general rather than one particular division. The change in religious attitude to life has definitely influenced my thinking regarding the essence and practice of medicine.

Introduction

Modern Medicine has made tremendous advances in diagnosis and treatment: in the time span of several decades more has been achieved than in centuries. Diseases previously incurable or deadly have become preventable or transformed into chronic, manageable ones or have become curable, either by medications or operations or a combination of various modalities.

However, many authors have described the deficiencies of modern medicine in the last two or three decades. First, the complexity of modern medicine mandates its practitioners to spend more and more time and effort on the practical aspects, leaving little time for personal interaction. This is undoubtedly the background for the so-called dehumanization of medicine, producing dissatisfaction in patients and subsequently in physicians and nurses as well. Second, although in the past the medical profession had very little to offer in terms of evidence-based cure and alleviation of symptoms, the doctor was highly regarded. On the other hand, modern medicine has cured or improved the lives of so many people, but its practitioners are increasingly regarded with suspicion about their professional capability or their financial or research incentives. Third, these and other factors have set the background for malpractice litigation, which has had a tremendous adverse impact on the status of the physician as perceived by both the public and the physicians themselves. Fourth, ensuing from previously described factors and others, there is burnout. Professionals providing various services, such as teachers, nurses and social workers are prone to burnout. However, modern physicians have evidently become much more prone to burnout than in the past. Modern medicine has become more biology-oriented, leaving little time and space for the emotional, social and value aspects of the patients - and their physicians.

The rise of modern medicine has been accompanied by a plethora of complimentary modes of medicine. According to some sources, for each doctor visit there is one or more visit to a complimentary practitioner. There appears to be a significant gap between documented evidence regarding the efficacy of various forms of complimentary medicine and the satisfaction professed by its users. Physicians tend to view complimentary medicine at best as a relatively safe outlet for those chronic problems (chronic fatigue syndrome, chronic back pain, or anxiety disorders) for which they do not have satisfactory solutions. At worst, they view complimentary medicine as charlatanism, where anyone can take a short or longer course in various unproven and obtuse practices, and set up shop without ever having had to prove proficiency as rigorously as they had to. Patients, on the other hand, turn increasingly to complimentary medicine to find remedies for their problems not addressed by modern medicine. Man is evidently *more* than the sum of his/her components, so abundantly and efficiently measured by modern medicine. It is probably this *additional* component that patients intuitively feel they have to have addressed. They need to have their physical ailments addressed and their rational thinking brain sends them to their conventional doctors. However, their *feeling* tells them there is something wanting with modern medicine and accordingly they seek answers in complimentary medicine, which may or may not answer that need. What complimentary medicine offers – as opposed to modern and often technical medicine – is an abundance of patient-practitioner interaction, often touching upon various emotional and psychological needs of the patient. Doctors in the past addressed these issues, but in the busy and often technical medical practice of the current era, time for these components has dwindled to barely detectable. Complimentary practices have stepped into the void. In addition, possibly, quite possibly, some of these modalities may offer actual cure or relief of medical problems way beyond the placebo effect with which modern physicians often and conveniently dismiss complimentary medicine.

Finally, there is a dimension of life and medicine beyond the biology, psychology and social networking of man. One may call this dimension a person's value system or spirituality, although the latter term may initially cause unease in some readers and definitely in practitioners of modern medicine. It is the purpose of this book to demonstrate this dimension both in theory and practice. Rather than discarding conventional medicine, the conscious embracement of the spiritual component supplements and empowers its achievements. These views are not original: they are grounded in millennia-old Jewish thinking. In some other religions there appears to be a concrete split between the mundane and spiritual, exemplified succinctly by Hermann Hesse in his classical novel Narziss and Goldmund, where the former is a monk, secluded from the real world, and the latter a real-world person and artist. In that view it seems to be either/or: either one lives a life in the real and physical world with all its passions, *or* one lives a life of the mind and soul, which requires withdrawal from (the pleasures) of physical life. On the other hand, Jewish thinking celebrates the real world as God's creation and, therefore, sees his purpose as demonstrating the spiritual presence in every aspect of life as we feel and experience it. It is man's challenge to appreciate the physical and expose the related spiritual dimension. By applying this thinking to modern medicine, one acknowledges its remarkable achievements *and* enhances its status and appeal to all those who recognize that man is more than the sum of his measurable components.

Many physicians have published articles and books with anecdotes about themselves or their patients. Several outstanding medical journals publish such vignettes, which usually serve to convey a message regarding the patient or the doctor. Family physicians and psychotherapists have discovered the tremendous therapeutic effect of requesting the patient to recount their life's story and major events and place, and associate their various ailments within the timeline and frame of these. Any individual's life's events are not random; they result from an interaction between a person's unique inner life and forces on the one hand and outside events on the other. Although significant surrounding events may have great impact on the individual, such as war, an epidemic or a tsunami, probably the vast majority of events in a person's life are the direct result of inner forces, mostly subconscious, which the individual expresses. The observant and introspective individual may, and perhaps should, derive important insights regarding himself by examining and analyzing the daily events of his life and definitely by taking stock at set periods. The physician, taking care of his patients and their illnesses, may have been trained to take care of their physical, emotional and/or social problems. It has definitely not been within the scope of modern medical schools to address the wider meaning of patients' illnesses. To provide a crude example: mechanics in car shops know everything about cars. They are able to diagnose cars' problems, take them apart, fix and make them functional. Nonetheless, all of us know that the car's value derives not from its physical make-up or its appearance. Rather, the car provides its owner the freedom to move about from place to place, meet people and attend events at distances beyond walking range. It often seems to me that patients and doctors are disgruntled with modern medicine in spite of its tremendous achievements, precisely because medical practice concerns itself with so many details of the human machine and has little time and thought to spare to address the *significance* of the patient's medical problems for the patient as an individual. I believe that there is a dire need to overcome this obstacle and supplement modern medicine with a dimension of spiritual relevance. The very term spiritual may cause frowning among physicians and patients: we are not accustomed to doctors being spiritual guides. In the past, doctors often provided such service, most likely because they did not have anything better to prescribe. Modern medicine has supplied physicians with many tools to help their patients and, consequently, the task of spiritual guidance has been relegated to rabbis or clergymen. Physicians need to reclaim part of their original profession. I believe that touching upon the wider significance of patients' illnesses serves the best interest of both the patient and the physician. Moreover, as the following stories demonstrate, this is possible, rewarding, and does not necessarily take much time.

This book is intended for both physicians and the general public and, accordingly, medical terms are kept to the minimal and/or are explained in lay language. The stories presented here are based on real cases, although identifying components have been fundamentally altered or fictionalized to protect the involved persons' privacy. Even if the author of this or any book or paper has particular objectives and intentions in mind, the reader will process the subject in his own unique way. Therefore, various readers may obtain different messages out of any book and this one is no exception. I would like to express the *hope* that this book touches the uniqueness in each reader and will encourage him or her to develop their own more spiritual approach to medicine, either as provider or recipient of medical care.

Chapter 1. Symptoms as symbols: The woman with the broken arm

It was ostentatiously a random accident. Lea Dowset, a 55 year old, married woman with four grown children, slipped in her bathroom and fell down hard, facing the floor. She knocked her face and some blood dripped from her upper front teeth, or maybe it was from her nose? She did not care about those few drops, as she was in excruciating pain. Her right upper arm had taken the brunt of the fall, its normally straight line was crooked and it was obviously broken. A subsequent radiogram revealed a compound fracture, which was straightened by an orthopedic surgeon and set in plaster of Paris. A careful check of her head did luckily not reveal significant trauma to soft tissue or bones.

But are any accidents random? Our rational mind makes us believe that there is no connection between evidently unrelated events, and that any attempt to associate between events which took place just before and after the accident is a dubious trick played by our psychology. However, in Lea's case three highly symbolic events will remain forever associated with this accident. The fall occurred on Passover evening, perhaps the most symbolic evening in the entire Jewish calendar. Jews all over the world gather, if possible within family context and celebrate the Exodus out of Egypt, lead by Moses, which occurred some three and one half millennia ago. The Bible describes the entire history in vivid detail: the circumstances leading up to the oppression and enslavement of the Jewish people, the miraculous plagues visited upon the Egyptians, the subsequent Exodus and crossing of the Red Sea and travels in the Sinai desert. The biblical story is permeated with symbolism and Sages over time have given multiple historical, psychological, spiritual and mystical explanations of most details. Lea's accident occurred two hours before onset of the Passover evening; she and her family intended to drive to another town to join her husband's family for the celebration. Relations with that family had always been cordial and close, so the fall was no obvious, subconscious loophole for not having to celebrate together.

A week earlier, Lea's mother had passed away at age 85. Her husband, Lea's father had died many years earlier of cancer. Like most widows, she never remarried, lived quietly and modestly by herself, until she developed Alzheimer's in her last three years and became more dependent and eventually lived with Lea's sister in Beer Shevah, a city in the south of Israel. Relations with this elder sister had always been complicated, although they reached a certain modus vivendi in the last few years.

One month before her death, her mother had slipped in the dark living room during one night and had broken her hip. Although successfully operated, she developed pneumonia and associated complications and never left the hospital. During the month of her hospitalization, Lea herself traveled south for several days in a row to stay with her mother, and returned to spend the weekends with her husband and children. One week before Lea's fall, her mother died and was buried in the town were she had lived, next to her husband. The ritual week of mourning was observed in Lea's sister's apartment and this was the first weekend after she came home. Although not religious, the very morning of her accident Lea had attended a religious service in the local synagogue, conducted especially to honor her mother. After its conclusion her husband observed that this was the first time in a long time that he saw her smile.

The signs of symbolism are abundant. But does that make them true? There is much epidemiological evidence showing that the incidence of serious illness, accidents and death is much higher among people who have lost close loved ones during the following year than among the general population. Modern, biological medicine has as yet to explain the mechanism of these various pathologies. It seems that mourning activates unconscious pathways, suppresses immunity and accelerates previously established disease processes. A bereaved person is possibly preoccupied by his loss, associated guilt and other feelings and consequently may be less careful of his health and even survival. Jewish mystical thinking suggests a strong association between one's inner and outer world; moreover, that one's inner world actually *produces* the circumstances and parameters of one's life. The quality of one's relations with one's spouse, family and place of employment are all determined by one's inner nature and the amount of emotional work one has invested to transform one's baser attributes into morally higher characteristics.

Ultimately, the significance of the accident and fracture of her right arm can only be worked out by Lea herself. However, the physician can set her on the highly-redeeming path of self-discovery. After diagnosis and taking care of the physical problems resulting from the accident, one could (and perhaps should, depending on the person's attitudes and requirements) point out the obvious symbolic circumstances. In Lea's case they include: the event occurring on Passover eve, one week after her mother's passing away, and the fact that her mother had sustained a fracture too as the initial event that ultimately lead to her death one month later.

According to quoted Jewish mystical writings, the real life is that of the soul, while the illusionary life is that of the physical world. This view, although radically opposed to that of western rationalism which itself is based on ancient Greek philosophy, holds that everything of *real* importance to a person happens within his mind and soul, while all things physical are transient and reflections of the soul. The real world serves as a décor, in which we are both actors and producers of the act. Becoming self-conscious leads to observation and introspection, which reveals who we are and what our true attributes consist of, in spite of romantic preconceptions, self loving and self-serving forgiveness. Except for a few chosen individuals, all of us need to act in the physical world, produce and participate in events, in order to create the very food for thought and self observation. If the latter leads to insight and change in attitude, verbal expression and behavior, the personal growth is usually obvious to oneself and the environment. Such a person is thankful to life and its circumstances and more readily acknowledges the supernatural. His life tends to become more tranquil and meaningful, and maybe less associated with traumatic events. The alternative is a barely consciously lived life, in which one apparently drifts from one random and meaningless event to the other.

Chapter 2. Making sense of suffering: The baby with end stage renal disease.

Joseph C. was born after a normal pregnancy and normal vaginal delivery, the second child of parents in their mid-late twenties of secular Sephardic background. His older brother was three years old and well. Joseph's growth and development were normal until he was about three months old, when his appetite decreased. He stopped gaining weight, he started to pass six to eight soft stools per day and he became irritable. The pediatrician initially thought that Joseph had milk allergy. However, routine blood tests revealed a much more serious condition: Joseph had severe kidney problems. An ultrasound revealed tiny, contracted kidneys, suggestive of end stage kidney disease. A renal biopsy was performed, without complications, and revealed scarred glomeruli, the tiny filtering units of the kidneys, indicating end stage renal disease unresponsive to drug therapy. A hemodialysis catheter was inserted into a large vein in Joseph's groin; three times each week Joseph was brought to the pediatric hemodialysis unit to undergo dialysis for several hours. His parents were devastated. The doctors, nurses and social worker were all very sensitive and supportive. Good relations were established between the parents and the staff. Hope was offered: once Joseph was two or three years old he would undergo kidney transplantation, either from a live, related donor, or from a cadaver. However, the intervening years would be demanding, very demanding. In addition to attending the dialysis unit thee times each week, Joseph would require constant attention to take care of his fluid and food intake, to give the necessary medications and to keep his intravenous line clean to prevent infection. The latter turned out to be the most challenging for his parents and would eventually lead to his death. Joseph developed recurrent blood stream infections with various bacteria and required frequent admissions to the pediatric department for intravenous antibiotic treatment, flush clogged dialysis lines and line replacement. With each complication his parents become more despondent and irritable. They were seen to quarrel, the father blaming the mother of possessing bad genes and inadequate care of the baby, the mother blaming the father for his inadequate emotional and physical support of the family. Breakup of the family seemed inevitable.

I met the baby and his parents as an infectious disease consultant during one of his admissions because of blood stream infection. It became immediately clear that his parents were at their wits' end. The mother had evidently cried and the father's face was tightly drawn. I shared with them the results of the blood cultures, the antimicrobial susceptibilities and need to change both antibiotics and the line, because of growth of fungi from the blood stream. I then suggested a book that I had read some time earlier that might help them cope with their terrible predicament, and they agreed, probably because they had nothing better to do. This book entitled "Many Lives, many Masters" was written by American psychiatrist Brian Weiss. He described himself as a straight psychiatrist, providing psychotherapy and medications, without religious or spiritual belief, at least until encountering the case he describes in his book. He writes about Kathryn, a young woman in her late twenties, who comes to see him because of depression. In spite of appropriate medication and psychotherapy over three years, her situation remains unabated. Then one day she comes to see him and tells a strange story. She and her husband had visited Chicago; they went to a museum, with a famous exhibition of life in ancient Egypt. The tour guide gave explanations next to each exhibit. Incredibly, Kathryn felt deep inside that the guide gave imprecise information regarding almost all exhibits. Being shy, and never having learned about ancient Egyptology, she did not say a word until privately after the conclusion of the tour. The guide took her to the museum's curator, who supported every single comment she made. With this information, the psychiatrist tried a new mode of therapy: hypnosis. Under hypnosis, he brought her back in time to ancient Egypt. Something remarkably happened: under hypnosis, Kathryn became more animated than he had ever seen her and she recounted remarkable details of her life as an ordinary woman until she died a traumatic death. During each subsequent hypnosis session, Kathryn went back to various other lives she had lived, all of which were sad and most ended with a traumatic death. Dr. Weiss did not know what to make of these reincarnation stories, but he was happy and astounded by the rapid progress his patient made. Kathryn became less depressive and happier after each session.

And then a story occurred within the story. During hypnosis, Kathryn reported that between one life and the next her soul was "somewhere", a place between places, with many souls and a Master. She then reported that the soul of Dr Weiss' infant son, who had died many years earlier, was out there and well. Dr. Weiss was flabbergasted. His first son, born during his final year in medical school, was born with a serious heart condition. He underwent several operations and eventually died only a few months old. He and his wife had been devastated. At the time he had deliberated between a career as pediatric cardiologist or psychiatrist, and the experience with his first child convinced him to choose psychiatry. He and his wife subsequently had several healthy children and they never again spoke about their firstborn, barely ever gave it a thought. Dr. Weiss wondered whether he unconsciously had transmitted evidence of this experience to his patient, but even so, he wondered how. What really made him reel, was when his patient, during a subsequent hypnosis, when again hovering in between two lives, told him that his baby son's soul wished to convey to his father that he was born in this world to carry out one short mission only: to help his father decide which professional direction to chose. Having completed that mission he could retire...

Joseph's parents were fascinated and obviously moved by the story. They were of traditional, but not particularly religious background and neither was I religious at the time. I told them the book was available at local bookstores, wished them all my best wishes and did not see them again. However, some five years later, while climbing the hospital's staircase, a woman in religious dress called my name. As I obviously did not recognize her, she reminded me of Joseph's case and the story I told them. They had bought the book, which totally changed their life. They understood that there was meaning in Joseph's disease and their suffering; that they had to open their hearts and minds, and start reading the super-text above events. They subsequently became religious, the marriage remained intact and she came to give birth to her fourth child. Joseph had become their blessing, who turned their life around from secular to deeply religious and spiritual.

Chapter 3: Futile medicine? The elderly, demented patient on the respirator.

Mr. Sarousy was 80 years, short of one week, when he was brought to the emergency department by one of his daughters. His wife had passed away about four years earlier and since then he had lived by himself. However, two years ago he sustained a stroke, which left him with left sided hemiplegia and inability to express himself verbally, although he was able to understand simple sentences and he recognized his children. For several months he stayed with one of his children, usually for several weeks at a row before being moved to another. Although he had seven children, four participated in this arrangement, while the other three were unable or unwilling to do so. Two days before admission, on the eve of Rosh HaShanah, the two-day Jewish New Year festival, Mr. Sarousy developed fever and cough. As he and the daughter he stayed with were orthodox the latter and her husband decided to wait and see rather than breaking the command of not driving on Shabath and festivals, although in case of a perceived threat the Jewish law actually obliges to break almost all commands in order to preserve and sanctify life. On the second day of the festival Mr. Sarousy deteriorated, his fever went up to $39^{0}C$ and he developed shortness of breath. In the evening, straight after conclusion of the festival, he was brought to the emergency department. The resident on call quickly made the diagnosis of pneumonia, put the patient on oxygen and initiated intravenous antibiotics.

The next day the causative organism, Streptococcus pneumoniae, was isolated from a blood culture. During the following two days the patient's respiratory condition deteriorated, his blood oxygen level dropped below 90 in spite of his oxygen mask and it seemed likely that he would tire and stop breathing. The attending physician and residents discussed whether this patient should be mechanically ventilated. On the one hand, pneumonia is an acute illness from which the patient could potentially recover and then be weaned from the ventilator. On the other hand, bleak statistics showed that less than one third of patients with pneumococcal pneumonia and bacteremia who require ventilation survive hospitalization. Moreover, this patient was already debilitated on account of stroke, completely dependant on others and had a poor quality of life. In order to discuss and solve this dilemma an urgent family consultation was called.

The meeting was conducted by Dr. Miller, the attending physician. Four of the children attended: two daughters with their husbands, all ultra-religious, the men in black suits and black hats, the women in long-sleeved dresses and wearing wigs. One additional daughter was non-religious, wearing jeans and one son attended, who appeared modern religious, with a knitted skullcap. Dr. Miller described the clinical situation of Mr. Sarousy, the pending respiratory failure, and the question whether to let nature follow its course and let the patient go, or rather insert a tube into Mr. Sarousy's throat and put him on a mechanical ventilator. The two ultraorthodox couples responded almost in concert, almost as if a reflex cord had been struck: of course everything had to be done to extend life, to sanctify life, even if the chance of survival was small, this was the dictum of the Halachah, Jewish religious law. The third daughter was much inclined to do nothing, rather than prolong her father's suffering by artificial means. The son wished to know more details: how much would his father suffer while being ventilated? The family expressed the wish to discuss the issue with the other family members and their rabbi. Not unexpectedly, Mr. Sarousy deteriorated that night and as no advance directives had been placed the resident on call intubated him and transferred him to a monitoring room in the medical department.

During the following days all seven children attended their father's bed. They split up amongst themselves and one of the children was present at all times, day and night. Mr. Sarousy did not improve, additional problems ensued, including central venous catheter associated bacteremia, acute kidney failure and decubitus ulcers. However, the patient received an intravenous medication to sedate and relieve anxiety. Days passed and the family became increasingly irritable. First, as often happens regarding seriously ill patients, they started to complain about various medical details: the machine beeped and the nurse did not quickly respond; blood pressure went up and down, should the doctor not pay more careful attention, etc. Subsequently, one of the non-religious sons started to quarrel with his religious sister, blaming her for her father's misery. "Look what your religious extremism has led you do, obviate the command to honor your father". Sleep deprivation, lack of adequate nutrition and disrupted family routines decreased inhibitions and hostile remarks among the siblings were traded at the patient's bed. Finally, two weeks after intubation, one of the religious son-in-laws vented his anger at Dr. Miller, blaming him for inadequate explanations at the initial decision making meeting and another son blamed him for conducting futile medicine, which led Dr. Miller to involve the department's chief, who invited all the family's members to his office on the next day.

All seven children attended: the two ultra-orthodox daughters, the secular daughter, the modern religious son, a modern religious daughter, and two sons, both with extensive tattoos on their arms. The chief expressed his sympathy regarding their father's illness as well as his high regard for their continued attendance at their father's bedside. Next, he requested the children to tell him a few, but most relevant details regarding their father's life. The modern orthodox son volunteered, and others joined in. The parents were born in Morocco, had immigrated to Israel during the mid 1950's during a large immigration wave. They had passed tent and barrack camps and then lived in two-room apartments. The father, although a successful shopkeeper in Casablanca, had worked in various manual jobs to make ends meet, while his wife raised the children. What sustained the father was his Synagogue attendance, three times a day and the occasional religious teachings he was able to pick up there. His children were his pride.

The chief expressed his appreciation for sharing privileged information. He wished to strengthen them with three comments. First, the family consisted of an entire spectrum of attitudes, like in most families. Accordingly, it would have been almost impossible for them to reach an agreed conclusion, even if Dr. Miller had put them through an entire course of end-of-life decision making issues. Second, the obvious question was not whether each or all of them wished to increase their father's chance to survive, but rather whether their father would have wished so. As he never had expressed any thoughts on this issue, one would assume that his religious attitude might have led him to do so, but this was speculation only. Finally, and most importantly, the chief expressed his belief that Mr. Sarousy was subconsciously presenting his children with a farewell present, the most precious possible. He gave them time. He announced his imminent death. He provided a set-up to convene all his offspring. Indeed, *after* his death all would convene too for observance of the seven-day shivah. However, the shivah days are hectic, each of the siblings receiving their respective friends and colleagues who come to console them. Meaningful talk among the siblings would be much limited. Therefore, their father, knowing that his children had developed into various contradictory directions, knowing that old frictions and rivalries prevented unity among his offspring, provided them with the most precious gift he could give them. He gave them time and the set-up to meet and talk, hopefully to defuse old tensions, in order to let them honor their father according to the fifth commandment prior to his death. By honoring their father at the end of his life, they would enrich their own lives and be more likely able to transmit their own hard-earned wisdom to the next generation. With due humility and respect the Chief wished the family much strength on the path ahead.

The conversation had lasted 15 minutes. The family left the office subdued, one or two with tears in their eyes. During the ensuing week, until Mr. Sarousy's death, no further friction was encountered between the family and the staff, or among the family members. The chief, who visited the shivah, encountered a healing family. Medicine, he knew, is not only biological-psychological-social; there is an inner, spiritual dimension and introducing it into the equation is healing for all concerned, including the doctor himself. Whereas biological medicine can be futile, completely integrated medicine, including referral to the inner dimension can *never* be futile.

Chapter 4: A hole in his heart

Endocarditis is an infection of the heart valves or adjacent membrane covering the inner aspect of the heart. It is an uncommon, but potentially lethal disease. It was first described by an eminent physician, Osler, in three landmark papers in the English medical journal The Lancet in 1885. Osler described the three cardinal symptoms, still called Osler's triad, consisting of unexplained fever, presence of a heart murmur and a cerebro-vascular accident or stroke. Osler's paper was based on an autopsy study: all of his patients had died. Indeed, in the pre-antibiotic era, starting with the introduction of penicillin into clinical medicine in the 1940s all patients with endocarditis perished. Currently, the annual incidence of endocarditis may be somewhat increasing. Fortunately, with appropriate antibiotic therapy, selected according to the susceptibility of the isolated organism the case fatality is less than ten percent. In addition, there may be residual morbidity due to complications, such as dislodgement and embolization of infected material from the heart valves with secondary obstruction of distant blood vessels such as the carotid arteries (leading to stroke) or arteries supplying blood to internal organs and limbs with catastrophic results. Most if not all bacteria causing endocarditis only infect heart valves that are deformed because of underlying pathology, such as prior rheumatic disease, a congenital abnormality or presence of an artificial heart valve.

Patients with endocarditis pose a formidable challenge to the internist and especially to the infectious disease consultant. First of all, while Osler described untreated patients who died, symptoms are nowadays often non-specific and usually consist of fever of several days' duration with accompanying malaise. As fever is a common manifestation of many different disease processes, the physician needs to possess a high index of suspicion to even consider the possibility of infective endocarditis. Second, physical signs may be very subtle and easy to overlook. Only if the doctor considers endocarditis among the diagnostic options will he or she order the specific tests that may confirm the diagnosis, such as blood cultures and a trans-esophageal echocardiogram. Third, these patients are usually seen first by their family physicians – and if fever continues antibiotics are often prescribed. Blood cultures are generally not obtained in ambulatory care prior to antibiotic use, which may reduce the chance to isolate the causative bacteria out of subsequently obtained blood cultures. Fourth, because the diagnosis is often elusive, case definition criteria have been developed, the so called Duke's University criteria. While these criteria are quite sensitive and specific most experienced infectious disease consultants have taken care of patients, who did not meet the case definition criteria, while no reasonable alternative diagnosis could be made. In such cases the doctor faces a serious dilemma: either "play it safe" by prescribing a four to six weeks' course of intravenous antibiotics - with possible associated complications; or follow through without treatment, running the described risks secondary to untreated endocarditis. Most physicians select the former option. However, blind treatment is hazardous without the identity and susceptibility of the causative organism firmly in hand.

Patients with infective endocarditis also pose a wide range of human challenges to the doctor. Upon learning the diagnosis patients often become quite anxious. Having an infection in one's heart sounds serious and actually may cause serious complications, even death. Moreover, presuming the causative organism has been identified, therapy usually consists of a combination of two or three antibiotics, almost invariably infused intravenously several times a day for four to six weeks. Even if the clinical course is otherwise unremarkable the inconvenience of such treatment is significant and disrupts the usual life pattern of most people. In some of the latter cases, one daily intravenous dose with one antibiotic drug is an option that may be given within the home setting. This regimen reduces inconvenience without compromising the overall outcome.

Over the course of my practice I have taken care of several hundred patients with endocarditis. Because of the associated anxiety and the prolonged course of the disease, a considerable investment in the patient-doctor relationship is called for and special relations often develop. Although the underlying infection is similar for most patients with endocarditis, each patient is unique and has specific clinical and personal features. I'll recount here the story of Meir Herat, one of my endocarditis patients with the longest follow-up. I met Meir when he was sixteen years old and I was doing my internship. Meir was referred to the hospital by his family physician because of a three week history of 38^0C fever, loss of appetite and two kilogram loss of weight. The family physician had carefully examined him and had observed an enlarged spleen. The only other abnormal finding had been a known heart murmur on account of a small congenital ventricular septal defect, which was unchanged since previous physical examinations. As several classmates had been diagnosed with infectious mononucleosis, the family doctor wished to rule out this possibility, but he was also concerned for endocarditis. Fortunately, no antibiotics had been prescribed –

and the three blood cultures that were obtained upon admission all turned positive within twenty four hours. The isolated organism, Streptococcus viridans colonizes the oral mucous membranes in large quantities and except for causing dental caries is otherwise quite innocuous. Teeth brushing often provide a route for these mouth bacteria to enter the blood stream, which usually remains unnoticed as the immune system removes these organisms within minutes. However, as described, these bacteria may infect previously deformed heart valves. Once Streptococcus viridans was isolated from Meir's blood cultures, the diagnosis of endocarditis was inevitable. Accordingly, a trans-thoracic echocardiogram was ordered; trans-esophageal echocardiography would become available only some ten years later. The echocardiogram revealed normal heart valves and a small vegetation that was attached to the known ventricular septal defect (VSD).

Treatment for Meir's condition consisted at that time of four weeks of intravenous penicillin, provided into six daily doses and in addition two weeks of three daily doses of intravenous gentamicin. The latter drug required frequently monitoring of blood levels to prevent kidney toxicity. This complicated regimen mandated hospitalization for the entire course of treatment. Fortunately, there were no complications and Meir was expected to attain complete cure. The attending physician had explained everything to Meir and his parents and they accepted the verdict. Nonetheless, Meir was somewhat upset, because he was preparing for the national chess championship as well as matriculation examinations in the exact sciences. He was a highly gifted student and had jumped two classes. His parents told me Meir did not need to prepare at all for his exams and was expected to pass with flying colors, but he was also very diligent and therefore wished to prepare just as all other students in his class.

During one of my daily visits with Meir, I requested permission to examine his mouth. I had read up about endocarditis, Streptococcus viridans and the association with dental problems. He appeared reluctant and, therefore, I explained the association between the mouth and the heart. When he finally opened his mouth I was astounded because of the widespread and extensive tooth decay. He admitted that there had been oral discomfort for quite some time, but he did not want to upset his parents. Dental care was expensive and he knew his parents were not well-off. Towards the conclusion of this hospitalization he was sent to the university dental student service, where one tooth was extracted, root canal treatment was started in two others and several caries were filled. Before discharge, the attending physician carefully explained to Meir and his parents the importance of twice yearly dental cleaning and examination, as well as the need for prophylaxis with antibiotics for most dental care. At that time, one big dose of penicillin was given orally within one hour prior to dental work and one dose six hours later. Such prophylaxis was expected to reduce the chance of blood stream invasion and heart valve infection. I had become quite attached to Meir: he had been battling a serious disease and he was only ten years my junior. I called him three months later regarding his matriculation exams, which he had passed and the chess championship, where he reached second place… "And please don't forget to take care of your teeth…"

Thirteen years later I was called as infectious disease consultant to see a young man with fever of unknown origin in the emergency department. I immediately recognized Meir's unusual family name, but I had difficulty recognizing the adolescent of many years ago in the tall, heavily built man in front of me. We met as old acquaintances, with smiles and handshakes and how have you been doing? Meir had completed two doctorates, in mathematics and physics, had completed a post doctorate in the US at a prestigious university and was doing high grade academic research. He had been exempted from army service on account of his VSD and past history of endocarditis. So what has brought you to hospital this time? It appeared a déjà vu situation: two weeks of fever, feeling tired, weak and without appetite. After ten days he had seen his long-standing family physician, who had obtained two blood cultures. That morning his family doctor had called him to inform that the blood cultures were positive and he referred Meir to the emergency department. The physical examination revealed the same loud heart murmur I recalled from the past, a moderately enlarged spleen and signs of small emboli in his conjunctiva and finger tips. When I asked permission to examine his mouth he grimaced, but agreed and I encountered an awful spectacle similar to the initial one on the previous admission. This time Meir underwent a trans-esophageal echocardiogram, which provides much greater details of the heart's inner structures. There was a large vegetation attached to the ventricular septal defect, but fortunately the valves were normal. The isolated organism, another Streptococcus belonging to the usual flora of the mouth was exquisitely susceptible to penicillin.

After Meir received the verdict (his term) of the second bout of endocarditis, he was upset even more than in the past. He was in the middle of time-dependent research projects. He needed to complete grant applications. And, he smiled sheepishly, he was dating a medical school student and was not yet sure he wanted to share his medical history with her at this point in time. So would he have to be incarcerated (again, his term) for a full month once more? I told Meir that new research had demonstrated that in his form of uncomplicated endocarditis one daily dose of intravenous ceftriaxone given for four weeks would be equally effective as the complicated regimen he had received in the past. Moreover, the major Health Maintenance Organizations (HMO) had organized the set-up for home intravenous treatment. Therefore, after receiving uneventfully several days of the antibiotic in hospital we could consider sending him home to complete treatment. Meir beamed. However, I told him we would probably not act according to this plan, because there was evidence of non-compliance. Meir's endocarditis had ensued most likely from serious dental neglect in spite of previous explanations and instructions. During the next several days Meir put up a serious effort to convince the attending team that he was fully responsible and could be relied upon. He would receive the weekly supply of antibiotic bags from the HMO and would infuse himself once daily. He would come to follow-up appointments as scheduled. And he promised he would take care of his teeth after completion of treatment for his endocarditis.

I saw Meir in the clinic at the conclusion of the one month intravenous antibiotic course. All signs of endocarditis had disappeared; the repeat echocardiogram revealed that the vegetation had shrunk considerably without clinical signs of embolization and repeat blood cultures were sterile. However, rather than being relieved Meir appeared depressed. His facial and body language exuded sullenness. Depression may be part of the symptoms of endocarditis; however, there had not been any sign of depression at the presentation of the infection and right now he was evidently cured. I wondered therefore about endogenous depression and accosted Meir directly. "How do you feel? You seem to be not too happy". He admitted feeling awful ever since being discharged from hospital. He had not told anyone about this new episode of endocarditis: not his parents or girlfriend, or his colleagues at the university. He had actually gone to work in the last two weeks, although he had carefully followed instructions regarding intravenous antibiotics. At work his thoughts had wandered and he had been unable to concentrate. He had lost all interest in his research. He just felt awful.

Whenever tensions and emotions run high, which occurs frequently in clinical medicine, I try to contain and defuse the issues. Rather than face the tension or emotion head on, I prefer to go circumspect. My intuition suggested a roundabout approach. "You know, Meir, I have always wondered about the possible source of your last name. Does Herat have a special meaning?" I had evidently kindled his interest. He looked up, his eyes somewhat brighter. "I have actually looked into it", he said, "when we had to write a project in high school on our family's origin. Initially I was embarrassed, because kids in the elite high school I attended were almost all of Ashkenazi (European) background, while I was from a Sephardic family. However, I learned that there was not too much to be ashamed of. My grandparents came to Israel from Afghanistan from the city of Herat, the second largest city in the country, located in the west near the Persian border. My father's paternal grandparents relocated from Isfahan in Persia to Herat. They had been wealthy merchants, dealing in carpets and jewelry and for financial as well as social reasons had made the move. There had been a large Jewish community in Herat and my grandparents had inherited the wealth and prominent social position of their parents. Israeli independence in 1948 led to a drastic change in attitude of the local population and the government toward the Jews in Afghanistan like in most Arab and Islamic countries and they had been forced to flee pennilessly. My grandfather actually adjusted rather quickly in Israel; he used his extensive business contacts to reestablish an "Iranian bazaar" that has been quite profitable".

Meir went quiet, evidently in thought. "Could you trust me, share with me your current thoughts?" He considered, then continued: "My parents evidently lost much of their inheritance because of the financial instability after the Yóm Kippur war and subsequent inflation. However, since then God bless things have picked up". Again some silence. "However, there is something else: something that tends to overwhelm me". He paused, swallowing something deeply emotional, perhaps tears. He resumed in a whisper: "You know, I have this hole in my heart".

There is no way of knowing what transpires in another man's heart. There are people who have tremendous problems that are obvious to the environment, such as financial or health problems. Some of these handle their problems almost with ease, as if there was no serious problem troubling their life. On the other hand there are people who are in great and perpetual emotional turmoil on account of minor issues. Of course I knew Meir had a ventricular septal defect from birth. He knew it was small and on account of its smallness there was no hemodynamic effect – and therefore there had never been a reason to send him for open heart surgery to close the tiny opening. Throughout his childhood he had always been handled with great care, as if he were fragile and in perpetual danger of falling ill or dying. He had compensated by intellectualization and rationalization, the only way of coping with the subtle messages he received from his environment, family, school and youth movement regarding a likely demise at young age. Endocarditis at age sixteen had reinforced his foreboding of dying young.

This time I would not give him a break. "I appreciate your trust and sharing with me these feelings" and waited to have him absorb my appreciation. "But how do you explain that rather than taking good care of your health, especially after your previous infection, that you choose to neglect your teeth". He silently pondered for several minutes. "You are right, you ask a good question. There are several answers, none too rational. First, I may have wanted to prove that I am stronger than the environment suggests, including the doctors. Second, I may have wanted to precipitate another infection in order to prove that I indeed am feeble and set to die young. Third, I eat tons of chocolate to neutralize the sourness in my mouth. Finally, possibly I let my teeth rot in order to feel physically the bitterness in my mouth which I feel deep down in my heart".

This rational, intellectual young man had superbly articulated his innermost feelings in a few sentences. When pushed against the wall by the circumstances of life, either disease or ordeal, the deeper layers of most people's souls open up like a flower petal in the sun. Great pain and emotion, buried under layers of cement, suddenly become accessible. Handled carefully, these newly tapped primal emotions may fuel a tremendous change for the positive, affecting all aspects of their lives, including their outlook of life, their relationships and their creativity. In view of the above I considered my next move. Of course I would have to convince him regarding psychotherapy. "What do you think made you depressed after the second bout of endocarditis?" He silently considered his answer. "I don't really know. Possibly I was upset that my previous calculation had not worked out. I was not stronger than the environment suggested. I actually could die young. Possibly, and quite likely I was upset and confused, because if this disease is so serious how come I am being sent home with only one intravenous antibiotic dose per day. Yes, I think I am confused and don't really know how to compose my feelings".

I warmly commended him for the superb emotional work he had done. "I strongly believe that this crisis in your life will serve as a turning point for the better. I suggest that you go work with a nice therapist to further explore and work through the important emotions and thoughts you have raised. I believe this will help you improve your feeling about yourself, your approach to your work, your success at work as well as the relationship with the people close to you. Of course I can provide you with names and phone numbers of therapists. And please don't forget about the dentist".

At the end of this visit Meir looked a different person. Rather than sullen and grey, there was new found energy in his face and physical demeanor. He seemed to look forward to this new direction of hope. He suddenly smiled. "I suddenly had a flashback. When I applied for a post doctorate in the US I had to type my name in many forms. You know what happens when you type my family name in the Word program? It automatically spell-checks and corrects my name from Herat to Heart. My last name actually consists of the same letters as heart. I used to see this as a verdict, as if doomed from birth. However, I am now inclined to see that miraculous circumstance as a suggestion. I have invested myself in mathematics and physics, i.e. my rational mind and I now need to spend time and energy on unknown emotional issues, things of the heart. You know, I actually look forward to it".

About fifteen years later a new technique was developed by ingenuous cardiologists and engineers. Until that time closure of septal defects required open heart surgery. The new technique involved an approach similar to cardiac catheterization: insertion of a thin tube through the femoral (groin) artery and threading it up to the left side of the heart. In case of coronary heart disease the tube is directed into the coronary arteries and contrast material is injected in order to detect presence and size of occlusions. The new technique allowed insertion of a stopper into the ventricular or atrial septal defect and attaching an occluding patch on both sides. Within several months these patches would completely become covered with endothelium, the membrane lining the inner aspect of the heart. There were no residual problems and so far no cases of endocarditis have been reported after successful occlusion of the septal defect. After our hospital had performed several of these procedures I decided to locate Meir and call him. Should I suggest he undergo this procedure?

The phone number I was able to find was from the Haifa area. The housekeeper answered: both doctors Herat were at work, would I like to leave a message? When Meir called me that evening he was obviously excited and appreciated my interest. Upon my question how he had been doing, could he please update me, he asked mischievously how much time I could spare him. When I reassured him he started straightaway. "When I left your office in the hallway I called the therapist you referred me to. For two years I did Jungian psychotherapy and I also attended several courses on symbol therapy and interpretation of dreams. Just consider the saying: taking things to heart. It is mindboggling: our language expresses symbolically how we feel and think about our body's organs. I actually *took* things to heart but over the years I have gained wonderful and liberating insights. I subsequently started a course in Kabala, which has transformed my life. After I married, my wife and I attended a course for people seeking their historical and cultural roots and we continue to be in regular contact. We moved to Haifa and I have been employed by a large petrochemical factory, where I am currently one of its chief scientists. My wife is a family physician". I heard him smirk and he added an afterthought as if to preempt a possible question: "She has nothing to do with congenital heart defects. We have three kids and all have healthy hearts. And so do I! Since my second bout of endocarditis I have taken good care of my teeth, dental cleaning every six months and I have not been in hospital ever since. I go to my cardiologist every year or two. Last year he suggested I go to Europe and undergo a trans-femoral artery closure of my VSD. I did, the procedure went well and there is no murmur anymore. You know, I first healed my heart in my mind and then the actual physical healing was but a minor issue".

Chapter 5: More futile medicine? Reading between the lines.

Sam Heiliger was a successful lawyer. He was born in England and educated at one of its choicest public, which means private, colleges as a barrister. After college he joined a law firm as a very junior partner, married and four children were born. While in his mid thirties he and his wife decided to immigrate to Israel. This was not an overnight decision. Both he and his wife were of modern-religious background and avid supporters of Israel. The question of immigration had been on their minds since their teenage years when they were members of a Zionist youth organization. However, growing career demands and family responsibilities made that youthful ideal a fading dream. When his law firm got caught in a financial crisis affecting England at the time and eventually went bankrupt, Sam was forced to spend time at home. He had never been in the habit of questioning God's ways, did not become depressed as many unemployed men are wont to do, but started looking for a new direction and job. His wife Cyril supported him emotionally throughout these months and it was Cyril who suggested the idea of immigration to Israel. During their boom years they had purchased a small apartment in Jerusalem, where they went for summer vacations; although the apartment was usually rented, as it happens it was currently free of occupants. After quite some thought and discussion, visits to the Israeli embassy and many other arrangements they moved to Israel. The first few months were spent at Hebrew language courses, after which the children were enrolled in their various kindergarten and primary school classes. Like many adult immigrants, Sam did not have an easy time to find a job. As planned, past savings helped them see through the first few months, but those funds were not expected to last much longer than one year. It was once again Cyril, who supported him emotionally through this period of self doubts and who helped him decide to set up a law office with a colleague, a more veteran immigrant from the USA. The building market was booming and they specialized in real estate, catering specifically to the large local Anglo-Saxon community as well as to foreign citizens, wishing to purchase a foothold in Israel.

I first met Sam some twenty years ago, when his firm was still quite new. I assisted a family member, living abroad but planning to immigrate in the near future, purchase an apartment in Jerusalem and Sam served as lawyer of the seller, an American immigrant himself. I was immediately taken by Sam's composed and dignified demeanor. He seemed the opposite of the sleek lawyer in bad clichés. He went thoroughly through the details of the contract, pointed out the relative advantages and disadvantages for each party. From Sam I learned the importance of reading *between the lines*, as well as looking for important things that might have been left out. Since those days, we have been in casual contact, usually because Sam needed some medical input regarding a client looking for legal advice regarding medical issues. He carefully refrained from medical malpractice cases, because he felt they might easily become debasing to himself and his client. When clients turned to him because of a medical grievance he preferred to run the case by me and subsequently directed his client for further medical or legal guidance. Financial gain was not his prime object; he wished to earn his living in God's world in an honorable way by providing his clients with the best possible advice that went beyond legal confines.

Now, twenty years after our first meeting, Sam arrived unannounced at my office. The night before his wife was admitted to the hospital after two days of fever and cough, and a large pneumonia was diagnosed. However, it appeared that Cyril had been seriously ill for three years, when she developed Alzheimer's disease in her late 50s. Like most of these unfortunate patients, during the initial months she was much aware that she deteriorated cognitively, which caused her much distress. However, Sam had always been able to reassure her by promising that he would continue to take care of her. He indeed made good on his word, when she lost all recognition of her family and became gradually wheelchair bound. He hired a nurse to stay with her during the day when he went to his job and at night he cared for her himself. We had spoken several times during these years, but, typically, he never even mentioned this personal tragedy.

Cyril rapidly approached respiratory failure and required intubation and mechanical ventilation. The question of refraining from "heroic measures" was never raised, not by the physicians or by the family. Cyril was after all only 62 years old, looked much younger than that and remained an elegant, dignified looking lady in spite of her disability. Antibiotics helped cure her pneumonia, but it appeared impossible to wean her of the ventilator and an opening needed to be made in her anterior neck to introduce a tracheal tube for continued ventilation. Like most similar cases, the prospect of surgery and creating an opening in the neck was met by revulsion and resistance by the family. A careful explanation helped reduce tensions: after all, a tracheostomy would help nurses clean the airway, would prevent development of a pressure sore and stricture in the trachea, and would actually improve chances of eventual weaning from the respirator. Moreover, if weaning was successful, the opening could be closed easily with only a tiny remaining scar. Sam and his children conferred during several emotional days and eventually agreed to the procedure. This was the first time I met their four children: young adults, in their late twenties and early thirties, expressing their concern for their mother's wellbeing with significant emotional involvement and intensity. They were all modern religious, wearing knitted skullcaps, decent young people raising their families, earning an honest living and making solid contributions to society. There was nothing philosophical about their attitude; they simply followed the fifth commandment, "honor thy father and thy mother". They expected and aimed at nothing less than their mother's recovery and her going back home, to be taken care of by their father and a nurse.

Sam and I had several significant conversations during the protracted hospitalization of his wife. The term "futile medicine" was never mentioned. Like at the time his first law firm went bankrupt, he never questioned why bad things happen to good people, or to him. His belief in God had been trusting and simple. However, he was concerned what would happen next. His children expected him to take his demented, ventilated and fully dependant wife home and care for her, just as he had done faithfully over the last few years prior to the recent deterioration. Just raising the option of a nursing home caused a serious emotional stir and Sam was determined to maintain harmony even at great personal and financial cost. Nonetheless, he was very much distressed.

To help him cope I suggested discussing two relevant biblical stories and their meaning. The first is the story of Cain and Abel, one of the first after the creation. "Abel became a shepherd, but Cain was a worker of the soil. In the course of time, Cain brought some fruit of the soil as an offering to God. Abel also brought an offering of the firstborn of his flock. God paid regard to Abel and his offering, but not to Cain and his offering. Cain became very angry and depressed. God said to Cain: "Why are you angry? Why are you depressed? Is this not so – if you improve, there is forgiveness, but if you do not improve, sin rests at the entrance. Its desire is unto you, but you can dominate it". Cain's soul was evidently of a high order; he after all discovered a way to get closer to God by making offerings, but nevertheless, God did not accept his. It is unclear from the biblical wording why God accepted Abel's offering but not Cain's. Commentators have suggested that Abel brought of the best of his flock and Cain possibly of less than optimal produce. Perhaps God preferred animal offerings above agricultural products? Whatever the reason, if that were the point of the story, the Bible would have told us. It seems therefore that the Bible does not wish to explain why things happen to people, although the Kabalistic literature has much to say about this. What appears much more important is what people do *after* things happen to them. That is why God told Cain to conquer his anger and depression, otherwise sinful action would follow, murder in his case. Rather, he should transform his strong emotions into a positive direction.

The second relevant Biblical story confirms the same idea. In Exodus (30:34-36, 7,8) is related the offering of incense: "The Lord said to Moses: Take yourself sweet spices, oil of myrrh, onycha and galbanum, together with clear frankincense, a light weight of each of these sweet spices. And you shall make it into incense, a perfume pure and holy blended by the perfumer, salted together". The Talmud (Kerithoth 6a) relates how and why incense for offering in the temple should be prepared. Rabbi Simeon son of Gamliel said: "The lye of Carsina *for what* was it employed? For rubbing on the onycha to refine its appearance." The Hebrew words "*for what*" can be vocalized in two ways, indicating two radically opposing meanings. One way would be "lamah", meaning why, which implies a backward look; while the other way of rendering the word would be "lemah", which means "for which purpose", indicating a forward look. As mentioned, the two stories indicate the same message: the Bible and Talmud are less interested in the reason things happen (although the Kabala delves deep into this issue), but rather focuses on what people do *after* these things happen. Do they become angry and depressed and turn to verbal or physical aggression; or do they turn these emotions around and direct these into constructive thought and behavior? Sam appreciated the relevance of our discussion and would share these ideas with his children.

During the next few weeks Sam, his children and their spouses divided the day and night time among themselves, so that one family member would be next to Cyril at all times. After Cyril was taken off sedative medications, she continued to sleep mostly, but intermittently opened her eyes. Sam felt her eyes indicated that she was occasionally conscious and aware of the presence of her family and events. He never felt comfortable to discuss her situation or plans for placement in front of her. Medical complications followed each other. Feeding was secured after placement of a percutaneous endoscopic gastrostomy tube, but she developed diarrhea. Most days Cyril had fever, ascribed variously to respiratory and urinary tract infections, deep venous inflammation and diarrhea. While Sam remained his calm and noble composition, his children grew discernibly tired, irritable and energy depleted.

Understanding for their parents' plight grew. Solutions were evidently going to be more complicated than simply "taking Mom home". I reminded Sam of a line he taught me many years ago: read between the lines. In their current situation the lines were ostentatiously mundane, such as physical inability; dementia; respiratory, urinary and fecal secretions; and placement. However, I urged him, read between the lines; better, read the super text, the highly personal meaning of the events. "Please", he begged me, "help me understand. I only see the misery of an impossible situation and how we are stuck as a family".

I reminded Sam of the Biblical Book of Esther, which is read twice at each Purim festival. The book tells the story of the Jews in Persia, some 2500 years ago, after the Babylonian exile. The capricious monarch of the time Ahashverosh dismisses his wife after a perceived sign of disobedience. After a lengthy selection process he marries a new wife, Esther, a Jewish beauty who is urged by her guardian Mordecai not to disclose her heritage. The king's grand vizier Haman, a proud, vain and cruel man, feels offended because all men bow before him, save Mordecai and sets up a plan to murder all Jews. Through a miraculous chain of events, things turn around, Haman is hung from the very gallows he erected for Mordecai, the latter replaces him as the king's second in command and the Jews are saved. While the Jews renew their commitment to their ancestral faith, it remains a fascinating fact of the Book of Esther that He who saved them is never mentioned or referred to. However, it is abundantly clear to the readers that Mordecai and Esther and the Jews knew that they had been saved by a miracle; they and the readers know that God was behind all these seemingly natural, mundane events. Tellingly, the title of the Book and its main hero's name, Esther, is in Hebrew exceedingly close to the word "Hesther", meaning hidden.

Life can be lived on two levels, the lower physical and the higher spiritual. Man cannot escape the physical dimensions of his life, the fact that he is earthbound and the very requirements of his nature. However, living one's life *only* in that sphere reduces Man to something much smaller than his potential offers. While some religions offer a choice between a mundane life in the world as opposed to a spiritual life of seclusion, Judaism celebrates life as God's creation and views his own role on earth the revealing of the spiritual in and above every single thing and event. Although I could point at some reading between and above the lines of Sam's family story, the task of revealing its meaning was ultimately his and that of his children's. I suggested to him that Cyril, unconsciously, perhaps at the behest of God, was transforming his family from a modern religious family living a very mundane life in the here and now, into a much deeper feeling and thinking unit. Events had precipitated much suffering and anguish, which had forced them to look and reach inside in a much deeper manner than they so far had been required to do. They had to look at their parents, their relationships and individual needs in a more nuanced way. Values such as mutual commitment, responsibility and family life were not taken any longer for granted and they felt tested to the core of their physical and spiritual being. Cyril, single handed, became the change agent, who transported this family from a secure, privileged modern-religious status to something higher and more spiritual.

As usual after talks with family members, I exchanged a few words with the attending physician, taking care of the relevant patient. Indeed, Cyril "did not go anywhere". She would never go back even to her abysmal state prior to admission. She would not regain cognitive functions, but would remain bedridden, permanently on mechanical ventilation and fed through a gastrostomy tube threaded through her skin into her stomach. But even in this tragic state, and especially because of it, she had been the change agent of her family, elevating them and bringing them into a closer contact with a higher level of significance of life.

Chapter 6. Perforated bowel: The unexpected benefit of a second opinion

Departments of emergency medicine and general surgery annually admit many patients with perforated intestines. The duodenum, the first part of the small intestine adjacent to the stomach, may perforate because of an ulcer or, less commonly, because of a tumor. Because microbial load is rather small in this part of the intestine, the risk of serious infectious complications is smaller and, provided corrective surgery was successful and the patient does not suffer from multiple other medical problems, the chance of survival and cure is quite high. On the other hand, perforations of the large bowel are worse by far. Common underlying illnesses include cancer of the colon, diverticulitis (an inflammatory condition of the colon common in people eating a western diet, low in fiber and rich in protein), and chronic constipation. Symptoms invariably consist of severe abdominal pain, with subsequently vomiting, fever and development of shock. Those lucky enough to come quickly to an emergency department often get diagnosed quite soon after admission. A plain abdominal radiogram usually shows free air, i.e., outside the confines of the intestine, indicating a leakage. The patient is quickly prepared for abdominal surgery, with intravenous fluids and antibiotics. During surgery, the surgeon removes fecal material from the abdominal cavity, determines the source of the perforation and creates a colostomy to let stool, coming from above flow into a bag attached to the skin. The perforation is closed, creating a "blind" distal loop. If and when the patient fully recuperates, the two parts of the intestine are stitched together during an elective operation usually after several months. However, the complication rate is often high on account of the massive amounts of bacteria in the abdominal cavity, in spite of cleaning and washing with antiseptic solutions during the initial operation. Peritonitis, massive infection within the abdomen, often leads to respiratory failure and need for protracted artificial ventilation and acute kidney failure, often with need for dialysis. Secondary infections develop frequently, including abscesses in the abdomen, which are diagnosed by ultrasound or CT-scan and are usually drained with tubes through the abdominal wall. Pneumonia, blood stream and fungal infections are common complications; therefore, infectious disease consultants are invariably on the team of physicians taking of patients with intestinal perforations.

Ms. Bluma Stavitsky was a 75-year obese woman, living with her husband in an ultra-orthodox neighborhood in Jerusalem. She suffered from diabetes and hypertension, both treated with oral medications for at least ten years, but was otherwise healthy and active. In the week before Rosh HaShana, the Jewish New Year, she developed constipation and abdominal pain, which gradually worsened during the 48 hours of the festival. In this particular year the Sabbath followed the festival, creating a 72 hour holy time, which is very taxing for every Jewish woman, who needs to prepare and serve many meals to usually large households. For Ms. Stavitsky it was inconceivable to desert her family on these days and to desecrate the holiness of the days by driving to a hospital. At the conclusion of the Sabbath, her son drove her to the emergency department. The admitting resident was alarmed by his patient's severe abdominal pain, quickly inserted an intravenous line, obtained blood tests, ordered intravenous fluids and obtained a plain abdominal radiogram. When, as expected, he saw evidence of free air in the abdomen, he called his attending surgeon and then called the operating room to announce the upcoming emergency operation. Ms. Bluma was relatively lucky. The perforation of her sigmoid colon was due to a burst diverticulum rather than to malignancy. However, there was quite some fecal material floating free in her abdomen, which was cleaned and washed with disinfectant. A proximal loop colostomy was created, the distal loop closed, and the patient was wheeled to the intensive care unit. During the next two weeks Ms. Stavitsky was treated with broad spectrum antibiotics and mechanical ventilation, but her kidney functions remained intact. Several abdominal abscesses were drained and out of the evacuated pus multidrug resistant organisms were isolated, including fungi. During the third week of the patient's stay in intensive care, she slowly started to recover, until a sudden high peak of fever indicated presence of a new infection. This turned out to be a fungal infection of the blood stream. At this point in time Mr. Stavitsky, the patient's eldest son demanded a second infectious disease consultation and his Rabbi told him to call me.

Second, third and even fourth opinions are commonplace in most hospitals. Some ethnic groups are more complacent and trust their doctors implicitly. Israelis are very health conscious and easily turn inquisitive whether their doctor is the most knowledgeable and competent around. When everything goes fine, they are thankful and often express their gratitude profusely. However, if things are serious or become complicated they may easily become critical. There is nothing wrong with second opinions. According to the best medical tradition, physicians of various disciplines and experience attend patients, especially the more complicated ones. Professionals often complement each other and bedside discussions often produce original ideas regarding differential diagnosis, tests and therapy. Therefore, in the more seriously ill cases additional experts in various fields have already been involved, often quite some time before families raise their request.. Accordingly, attending physicians may feel criticized or even accused of not providing the best possible care. This may especially be the case if the requested expert consultant is based in another hospital. I have received numerous requests to see patients in other hospitals, but have rarely done so. I prefer to explain to the requesting family member that his patient is in an excellent hospital, which sports an excellent infectious disease unit with competent infectious disease consultants, which is the situation in the vast majority of hospitals. Rather than spend a considerable sum to induce a consultant to visit another hospital, in order to pay for his time and effort, I try to convince them to seek contact with the infectious disease consultant already involved, or at most request a second opinion from the chief of the particular service. This is less expensive, does not shuffle sensitive feathers as much and more likely leads to continuity of care.

Upon receiving the request to see Ms. Stavitsky I discussed the case with the infectious disease consultant already involved. As in most of these cases, it did not seem to me likely I would have some brilliant new insight regarding diagnosis or therapy. I examined the patient, saw all recently performed imaging tests, reviewed her laboratory tests and spoke with the attending physician in the intensive care unit. Ms. Stavitsky obviously had multiple infections, including residual ventilator pneumonia; intra-abdominal abscesses, which had been adequately drained while antibiotics took care of the remaining infection; and most likely a fungal infection in her blood stream. All tubing had been replaced, including intravenous lines. Antibiotics had been adjusted to cover all isolated organisms and other pathogens likely to be involved. I had only minor new recommendations to the treating team and, with nothing better to do, I invited Ms. Stavitsky's son for an in-depth conversation and explanation about the situation. Mr. Stavitsky heard my carefully reasoned explanations, which I presented without technical language and in terms easily understandable by non-professionals. When I reached the bottom-line that everything reasonable and necessary was done and that his mother received the best possible care to ensure recovery and survival, he simply exploded in my face. All the worry, fatigue and frustration accrued over two weeks of intensive care treatment, and lack of certainty regarding his mother's future, he expressed in a torrent of verbal abuse and anger, accompanied by ample hand and arm gesturing.

I teach my residents that the angrier and louder patients or their families become the more silent and humble we physicians need to become. Their anger, after all, has nothing to do with the treating physicians, and everything with their own pain and frustration. We serve as their wailing wall. Although we never promised to cure all patients, we expect of ourselves (and so do our patients) that we spend our best in professionalism and time to assure the optimal outcome for our patients. Indeed, if patients do not recover or develop complications, we are frustrated ourselves, which not necessarily means that we deserve to be on the receiving end of their anger. It is evidently part of our job to ventilate our patients and their families. However, rather than silently undergo the torrent of their raw anger and frustration, we could and should try to reframe the issue and direct their feelings into a more positive direction. Quietly I invited Mr. Stavitsky to join me on the small walk to the toilet. Next to the outside sink hang a framed plaque with the blessing which religious Jews recite after use of the bathroom. I asked him to read the blessing. He turned even more vehemently angry: "You, not even wearing a black skullcap like I do, want to teach me the meaning of a blessing!" I insisted: "Please, do me this favor and read it". So he did: "Blessed are You, Lord our God, King of the universe. With wisdom You have formed man, creating within channels and passages innumerable. In Your sublimity, You know that were they torn or obstructed we could not survive and stand before you even one hour. Blessed are You, Lord, who works the miracle of healing all flesh". I repeated and accentuated after him: "Channels and passages. Were they *torn* or obstructed, we could not survive even one hour". And I added: "You have recited this blessing for all your life maybe five or seven times a day. And it refers to what your mother suffers from right now". Over the next minute or so his anger subsided, the redness of his face subsided and he turned into a calm and kind man he probably always was. "Thank you", he managed to mumble. "You have taught me something. You doctors have kept my mother alive for several weeks longer than God's plan. Please keep doing the best you can to help her completely recover. I'll keep praying for God's blessing of your efforts".

Not unexpectedly, Ms. Stavitsky died from a general fungal infection and multi system failure. I did not attend the funeral, or the *shivah*, the seven-day mourning period. I probably did not feel very comfortable to enter an ultra-religious family's home. Maybe I did not want to upset her son after his emotional outburst, making him feel ashamed when encountering the very doctor who "has taught him something". However, several weeks later I received a letter from this very son, in which he thanked me, other doctors and nurses for doing our best to take care of his mother. It was not in our ability to help his mother recover; however, his mother's final illness helped her son reach an inner depth that evidently so far had not been accessible to him. Could that perhaps have been her farewell present?

Chapter 7: CMV: Counseling with wisdom in the face of uncertainty.

Ill young women often generate much discernable concern and emotion among their doctors. Young women are the focus of their families, in Hebrew the "chief of the household" and a serious illness affecting their wellbeing or survival poses an existential threat to their entire family. Somehow, the concern we feel or should feel for each patient is augmented and becomes more palpable. Possibly we are able to identify more readily with the young female patient and her family, or perhaps our sense of protectiveness is activated. If the ill woman is pregnant concern and emotions only increase.

Over the years many concerned young couples have come to my infectious disease clinic for a consultation or second opinion regarding possible infection during their pregnancy. The classic TORCH acronym indicates the most frequent culprits: TOxoplasmosis, Rubella, Cytomegalovirus, Herpes virus. However, there are many more organisms that may cause damage to embryos and pregnant women, including syphilis, which during centuries - until the advent of penicillin in the 1940s - has caused terrible suffering and deaths with associated psychological and social impact. With the development of an effective vaccine against rubella, provided to young children (and adult women whose blood test shows that they are not immune), this virus has almost completely disappeared as cause of trouble or concern to pregnant women. Its place has been taken by cytomegalovirus, or CMV. This virus and the closely related Epstein-Barr virus, or EBV, are common causes of a minor viral disease in young children. As recent as the 1970s, up to 80% of army recruits, supposedly representative of young adults had protective antibodies for CMV and EBV, indicating that they had been exposed to these viruses in the course of their lifetime. Infection occurs through close contact and, accordingly infection occurs usually in toddlers or young children, where it often manifests as a mild febrile illness of short duration. With increasing quality of life, improved hygienic conditions and development of smaller families, more people reach adulthood without prior exposure to these viruses. Currently, in many countries more than 50% of young adults do not have serologic evidence of immunity to these viruses. Young adults may become infected in college dormitories, army training, or when dating, hence the term "kissing disease" for the condition known medically as infectious mononucleosis. In young adults this disease may be asymptomatic, but more often manifests with significant fever, malaise, lack of appetite and weakness. On physical examination the lymph nodes, liver and spleen may be enlarged. Blood tests usually show an increased lymphocyte white blood count and elevated liver function tests, while the diagnosis is usually confirmed with serologic tests demonstrating specific antibodies, immunoglobulin M (IgM) and immunoglobulin G (IgG). A positive IgM antibody test for CMV together with a negative IgG test in a patient with an acute febrile illness, usually indicates acute CMV. However, presence of IgG antibody for CMV and negative IgM indicates past exposure, while it is often impossible to determine when this past exposure occurred, either recently or in the distant past. Presence of both IgM and IgG may indicate recent infection, because IgM is the first antibody to appear, to subsequently disappear – usually within a few weeks after the acute infection – to make place for IgG which remains life-long and provides protection against re-infection. There are, however, instances when IgM may reappear in people who have become immune against CMV in the past and consequently are IgG positive - as we shall see below.

Gynecologists and obstetricians following pregnant women conduct routine tests at certain points in time during the pregnancies. No country has introduced routine testing for CMV. However, in the current age when malpractice suits have become common and a frequent outlet for patients' frustrations regarding undesired outcome of their disease, hospitalization, procedure or pregnancy, or the most certain route for obtaining financial compensation, many obstetricians obtain routine serologic tests for CMV during pregnancy. They do so, because previously non-immune women may contract CMV during pregnancy, which may lead to congenital illness of the newborn. Primary CMV in pregnancy usually manifests as an acute febrile illness as previously described for adults. It also may be asymptomatic, although this is evidently much less common in adults than in young children. Primary infection in pregnant women, whether symptomatic or not, is accompanied by infection of the fetus in some 40-60% of cases, which can be demonstrated by isolating CMV from the newborn babies. Infected babies are fortunately asymptomatic in up to 90% of the cases; however, they may suffer from several symptoms, ranging from various degrees of nerve deafness to devastating neurological malformations. Obstetricians fear adverse outcomes of pregnancies, including congenital CMV, as they may become the easy target of accusations or worse. Malpractice trials focusing on congenital CMV have been conducted and won against obstetricians, who failed to diagnose the infection or provide appropriate counseling.

Shaul Plotkin and his wife Hanna came to see me with a pile of routine test results conducted during Hanna's current pregnancy. They were Hassidic, ultraorthodox Jews in their early twenties. They had been married four years and had a healthy two year old son. Hanna's current pregnancy was so far uneventful, until a routine blood test performed by their doctor during her tenth week of pregnancy, showed positive IgM and IgG for CMV. For interpretation and counseling their doctor referred the couple to the infectious disease clinic. Hanna did not recall any febrile illness during her current pregnancy; however, their son who attended a day care center had had several upper respiratory tract infections. Other blood tests Hanna had done did not reveal any sign of acute infection. We reviewed the test results and discussed the situation at length. First, we talked about the possible implications of primary CMV in pregnancy, which brought Hanna close to tears. Second, what was the evidence that Hanna indeed had primary CMV? Could she have had CMV in the past, with development of protective IgG antibodies and the current appearance of IgM antibodies were just a sign of the irregularity of her immune system on account of the pregnancy? Was it possible to determine the date she first encountered CMV? In fact, there were two options, both to be explored, to try and determine whether Hanna had been immune prior to the current pregnancy. The first way was to request a specific blood test, CMV avidity, a laboratory phenomenon, which if highly reactive would indicate that the primary infection had occurred three months or more in the past, i.e., prior to her current pregnancy. However, the other way could and did prove even more helpful: see if their health maintenance organization had laboratory proof of a positive past CMV-IgG antibody for Hanna. I called her family physician, who checked Hanna's laboratory file and found that two and one half years earlier, most likely during her first pregnancy the CMV IgG and IgM had also been positive. The subsequently performed avidity test, although unnecessary, turned to be highly reactive, as expected. This couple was lucky, although they were definitely rendered anxious for several days by their obstetrician, who had requested an unnecessary blood test. Too relieved, they would definitely not resort to making complaints.

Mordecai and Esther Mizrachi were not so lucky. They were a secular couple in their late twenties, Mordecai an engineer and his wife a high school teacher of mathematics. They had two healthy daughters, age five and three. The current pregnancy had been uneventful until the routine blood test for CMV in her eighth week of pregnancy came back, showing a positive IgM and IgG, just like with the Plotkin couple. The phone call to her doctor showed that a blood test for CMV during her prior pregnancy had been negative: both IgG and IgM were negative. With these data I knew the discussion was going to be more painful. Esther had evidently had primary CMV between the last and current pregnancy and it might turn out impossible to know when this had transpired. After reviewing the clinical aspects of CMV, chance of primary versus recent infection and associated risks, we reached the bottom line: the recommendation for the CMV avidity test. If avidity was high, this probably indicated that infection had occurred prior to the current pregnancy, which significantly decreased the risk that the fetus had become infected and ill. If the avidity was low or borderline, this suggested more recent infection with associated risk for the fetus. Would they prefer to do the test and come back to discuss the implications, or would they prefer to discuss these upfront? Perhaps because of their scientific and rational backgrounds, both wished to discuss everything here and now.

I warned them that this was going to be the unpleasant part of our talk. This having said, I wished to strengthen them by applauding their mature and reasoned approach to this challenge to their young family. I would provide the medical information and they would decide using their own values. So, if the avidity came back low or borderline, this would likely indicate primary infection during pregnancy. The chance of infection of the baby was 40-60%, with the chance of symptomatic infection about ten percent. Esther quickly calculated that the baby had therefore a chance of at most about 6% to be symptomatically ill. I responded that the statistics were unfortunately not that definite, but her estimation was probably as close as one could get. With otherwise normal pregnancies there is a 1-2 percent chance of congenital malformations; therefore, concluded Mordecai, with primary CMV the risks were perhaps six times as much. They essentially had three options. First, they could opt for a first trimester termination of pregnancy, which could be performed with oral medications and/or dilatation and curettage. The eyes of Esther, not withstanding her calm and reasoned demeanor, rapidly filled with tears, indicating how upset she was. Mordecai responded marvelously; he turned tenderly towards his wife and put a protective arm around her shoulders. "We will do nothing", he said, "unless you are in entire agreement, including the deepest recesses of your feelings". The second option, I continued, involved waiting until the twentieth week of pregnancy, when enough amniotic fluid had accumulated around the baby to allow for obtainment of a fluid sample by inserting a small needle through Esther's abdominal wall into the uterus. This sample could be rapidly tested for presence of CMV. This time Mordecai interrupted: "Did you not say that the baby is likely to be infected with a small chance only of being ill? I confirmed his question. Indeed, the fluid could be positive, indicating infection, which would not determine whether the baby was ill. "So what", he said, "if it is negative you are really relieved. However, what do you do with the result if it is positive?" I appreciated their quick understanding of the emotionally charged information. I was used to repeating various components of the explanations. Here I just could continue, step by step. In the case of suspected primary CMV one conducts an amniocentesis not for reassurance; although the involved risk is very small, perhaps one in 1000 instances leads to a serious infection of the amniotic fluid, which almost always leads to rapid termination of the pregnancy and often death of the fetus and may lead to significant morbidity of the mother. It is, therefore, sensible to do an amniocentesis if diagnosis of CMV infection has practical implications, i.e. discontinuation of pregnancy. Doing an amniocentesis for reassurance only is perhaps not justified, considering the small, but serious risk of infection. Mordecai had never heard of a second trimester interruption of pregnancy. "Is that done as a first trimester pregnancy", he wished to know. No, I said, if a first trimester interruption is physically and emotionally unpleasant, a second trimester interruption is worse. It involves introducing a lethal solution into the uterus, which starts contracting and precipitating the process of birthing, eventually leading to expulsion of the uterus' non vital content. Esther's face had turned ashen. Once again Mordecai quietly put an arm around her shoulders. Once she recollected her feelings, she briefly whispered that she could never do such a thing.

This lead to the third option: "Do you remember I mentioned a third option?" This would entail doing nothing. Each healthy new baby is a miracle and as mentioned there is always a small chance of medical problems, quite a few of which can be corrected or improved with modern medicine. The chance of serious symptoms with CMV is quite small, so one could opt for doing nothing, perhaps pray and hope for the best. The obvious question they needed to ask themselves was, whether they would have the emotional and social resources to deal with a possibly ill baby. Would the coping with adversity and illness strengthen their commitment to each other and their family, or would it tear them apart? "What and how do other people decide", they wished to know. They knew I see many couples with this conundrum. I told them that there are three stereotypical approaches. The first involves the ultraorthodox religious: most Rabbis in that sector are totally opposed to interruption of a pregnancy for primary CMV infection, although the Halachah, the Code of Conduct of Judaism certainly allows so. However, if there is any danger to the mother on account of the pregnancy, almost all Rabbis concur that it should be interrupted. The second stereotype approach, which I encounter only rarely, is that of the most mundane, down-to-earth people, who wish to proceed with each pregnancy only if they are close to one hundred percent certain regarding the positive outcome. The third approach is the most common and involves modern religious and secular people. They weigh the medical evidence and preferably do some significant soul searching. The couple discusses the pro's and con's of each step and option. I told Esther and Mordecai that any of these options they choose would be acceptable by the Halacha and the country's laws.

On a more personal level, I wished to strengthen them by three comments. First, during all subsequent pregnancies they would not need to worry about CMV anymore, as Esther was already immune and immunity lasted lifelong. Second, parenthood involves lifelong responsibility and commitment. I wished to underline that comment by telling them the anecdote of an elderly man asking his rabbi until which age one should be anxious about his children's wellbeing. The rabbi answered "until age 65", which produced an audible thigh of relief from the man. When the rabbi wished to know why the man appeared so comforted, he said he would turn 65 the next day, upon which the rabbi said that he intended that it is age 65 of the children before an elder may discontinue to worry…. Mordecai and Esther smiled. They knew they joined the club of all those parents, who wish and work tirelessly for the health and benefit of their children and pray for the best possible outcome.

"And my third comment?" they wished to know. In a way this would reinforce the second comment. Mordecai and Esther faced together a serious challenge. They had to decide for the wellbeing of their baby and future of their family. They had to evaluate the strength of their relationship. Every marriage faces crisis times. One could question the fairness of life's problems, "why bad things happen to good people" and I referred them to the eponymous book by Harold Kushner. This is essentially a non starter, because no one is going to provide a reasonable response. Rather, what determines is what people do when things happen to do them. Do they become depressed, aggressive or abusive? Or do they rally to each other's support? The vast majority of people do cope well with their problems, they consult their families and friends, they delve down inside their inner selves and often detect emotional and spiritual resources they never were aware of. People grow by facing life's problems. I said I knew they were not openly religious. Nonetheless, I referred them to the well known biblical story of our ancestor Abraham, the first Jew.

According to the Talmud, the oral law, Abraham was tested ten times and each time he wrestled, overcame his tests and matured. The Hebrew word for challenge ("nysayon") indicates test, but also banner and also miracle. Therefore, a test essentially invites and induces one to rise to the occasion and grow through the process. An untested person does not really know who he is. Although we would wish and pray for a quiet life without undue challenges, it is exactly the coping with those challenges which helps us expose and develop those very qualities buried inside which we never knew of. A person who was tested and faced his challenge successfully is never going to be the same. He is and knows himself to be richer and wiser beyond recognition. In a sense, Life sensed that Mordecai and Esther were ready for a challenge and presented them with the question of primary CMV in pregnancy. Their task was cut out: they needed to decide what was best for their baby and family, but through this process they needed to assess the quality and strength of their marriage. Whatever their eventual decision, they would grow and enrich throughout the process.

Several days later they sent the result of CMV avidity, which was borderline positive and therefore not helpful although probably indicating recent CMV infection. I called Mordecai to know whether they had reached a decision. They had not, but amniocentesis and termination of pregnancy at week twenty of pregnancy was out of the question. They deliberated whether to continue or terminate now, but he wished to thank me for the stimulating conclusion of this most difficult doctor's visit. I am vain enough to appreciate these comments of appreciation. More to the point, I feel that I have done my duty as physician, that I have taken care of the biomedical problem of my patients, but also have addressed the involved emotional, social and spiritual dimensions.

About seven months later, Mordecai called me through the hospital's telephone operator. He wished to invite me for the Brith Milah, the ritual circumcision, of their son, who was born about four weeks earlier. There had been a transient problem of low platelet counts on account of congenital CMV infection, which is why the circumcision was postponed, but there were no other signs of disease. Unfortunately I needed to decline on account of a prior commitment. However, some three years later the couple with their son came to my office without prior appointment, the boy sporting a hearing aid behind each ear. They had just come from another visit to the child development center. He functioned entirely normal and spoke well as expected for a child his age. Seeing the hearing aids, my first, gut response had been one of anxiety: where they going to accuse me? Filing a malpractice complaint? Of course I could not remember the details of that one clinic visit, although I make careful notes in the clinic files. Had I really left the decision making process open for them? Had I seduced them into continuing the pregnancy? However, the parents' faces were relaxed and happy. They wished to keep me abreast of the wonderful developments in their marital relationship, personal and family life and they ascribed all these positive developments to the special son they had been blessed with and the circumstances of his birth. They knew all of them had grown marvelously and miraculously through the experience. And by the way, Esther is pregnant again: is there anything special they needed to do or follow through regarding CMV?

Chapter 8: Sexually transmitted infection: fertile ground for personal development.

Sex obviously fascinates the human mind from the moment we enter puberty and the body develops sexual feelings. During adolescence, subsequent psycho-social development and marriage people ideally learn how to express their sexuality appropriately within the framework of a meaningful and lasting relationship. Nonetheless, sexual thoughts and fantasies continue to flash through the minds of many people, either precipitated by encounters with attractive people or just out of nowhere. Some people cherish these fantasies, other abhor those thoughts and would wish to abolish all of it. However, there is a vast distance between fantasies and the actual carrying out of sexual fantasies in normative people. Inhibitions play an important role: the fear of unwanted pregnancy, the fear of catching a disease and the fear of being caught in case of adultery with associated implications for relationships. However, there may and ideally should also be positive factors that should help control sexuality and transform it into a constructive force. Such force should help balance between sexuality within the context of a lasting, loving and creative relationship on the one hand, and spiritual growth on the other hand, as we shall subsequently see.

During my fellowship in infectious diseases in a large US city the fellows were required to spend one afternoon each week in the sexually transmitted disease (STD) clinic run by the local county Health Department. Attendees were mostly young and underprivileged citizens living in inner city locations and most lacked medical insurance, although an occasional well-to-do middle class gentleman would turn up who preferred not to see his own family doctor with his embarrassing problem. After hearing the patient's complaint, we were instructed to administer a standard questionnaire. We fellows were in our early to mid thirties and felt quite mature, but we were proven naïve when we heard that many of our patients had had up to ten different partners in the last month before their visit and many had had many more in the previous half year. In addition, we learned of sexual practices we had never heard about. Most of us fellows loved the experience: within several hours we took care of several patients with gonococcal or non-specific urethritis, syphilis in various stages, genital warts and occasionally more uncommon sexually transmitted infections. We did the pelvic examinations to diagnose pelvic inflammatory disease in women. However, the one thing which really overshadowed the enthusiasm of working at the clinic was the need to tell young people that the HIV test, obtained with their permission at their initial visit one or two weeks earlier, had come back positive. This was the era before highly active anti-retroviral treatment (HAART) became available, which has turned HIV into a chronic and manageable disease that possibly does not reduce normal life expectancy. At that time we had to inform a young person that he or she had a devastating disease that would kill them at most within a few years. These encounters were heart rending. We fellows used these terrible experiences to stimulate the other patients to more careful behavior. After we examined the patient and took their laboratory tests to the small lab on the premises, a formidable public health representative entered the room in order to obtain lists of names and addresses of sexual contacts to be subsequently tracked down and treated. Only after this encounter did we return to the patient, provided treatment and tried to engage the patient in an educative discussion regarding subsequent sexual behavior. From the beginning of my medical career I have always felt grateful that patients were willing to share with me their medical and personal sorrows, a thankfulness that has not diminished with time. I am not sure whether all or many other doctors consider this a privilege; after all, they studied and worked hard to acquire the knowledge and experience to help sick people. I consider myself like the patient in front of me and feel lucky not to have contracted the disease they have. Moreover, I feel thankful not to have the obsessive, compulsive or various other inclinations that lead to dangerous practices such as casual sex, promiscuity, overeating and drinking or drug abuse. Work in that STD clinic reinforced my personal appreciation and reinforced my commitment to a mutually monogamous relationship with my wife. It also helped me develop a (hopefully) non-condescending attitude to my patients, in which I try to provide counseling appropriate to their attitudes. For example, I learned it was useless to preach the value of a mutually monogamous relationship in adolescents and young adults, who had ten or more different partners in the last month or so. Rather, I suggested that fear of a new STD and especially HIV should serve to decrease the number of sexual partners and always use a condom.

During the last few months of my fellowship I wrote a blueprint for the new infectious disease unit which I would try to develop after returning home. On my to-do list was definitely a walk-in STD clinic. However, visits with more experienced directors of infectious diseases units throughout Israel quickly opened my eyes regarding this idea. First of all, all Israeli citizens have medical insurance and, accordingly, upon developing an STD most would see their family physician.

Second, Israel does not have inner city populations the way the US has. Individual cases of promiscuity, homosexuality and drug abuse exist here as elsewhere, but, in case of a medical contingency, these people like other Israeli citizens could easily turn to a variety of caregivers, including the local emergency department, community based outpatient clinics and their family physician. Third, the Israeli public prefers to attend an innocuously called infectious disease clinic rather than an entity explicitly called sexually transmitted diseases clinic. I learned from my more experienced colleagues and refrained from opening an STD clinic, although since then both in Tel Aviv and Haifa STD clinics have opened, catering to a less settled public. For my part, I see patients with STDs in the infectious disease clinic, the medical emergency department and upon request from a gynecologist in the gynecology clinic.

Amnon Davidson was a twenty one year old yeshiva student in a black skullcap, no beard or side locks and accordingly I could easily classify him as being ultraorthodox, or Haredy and definitely not as Hassidic, because the latter never shave their beards and grow side locks. He came to see me in clinic because of a dream. Ever since he had this dream about two weeks earlier he was in tremendous anxiety, could not concentrate on his studies and lost his appetite. Did he see his family doctor? No, he had not and he was quite anxious that I should not involve his doctor. Had he discussed his dream with his Rabbi, a study friend, or his parents? No, he had not, could and would not, but he had finally gathered enough courage to come to see me. Evidently he had learned that in my hospital, officially observant of the Jewish Halachah (law), there were medical services operating according to the Halachah that dealt with sexuality and fertility such as the in vitro fertilization (IVF) clinic, genetic counseling for young religious people prior to onset of dating, as well as the infectious disease clinic. His dream involved an attempted sexual encounter with a young woman. The dream encounter took place in the local synagogue in the women's section after Shabbat morning prayers and everyone had left. Did Jacob know the woman? His answer was negative, but not quickly and natural enough to convince me, but I was wise enough not to probe any further. I asked what had brought him to me as infectious disease doctor. If the presence of sexual dreams concerned him, perhaps a wise Rabbi could provide guidance? However, he was too embarrassed to ask a rabbi. Moreover, his face flushed and his voice now hoarse, he whispered that he was concerned that he had become infected with HIV.

I was astounded! What a huge contrast between the world-wise inner city population that I had encountered in the STD clinic and the innocence of this young yeshiva student! However, after a second my initial surprise made place for suspicion. Perhaps this young man had had a real life encounter and fabricated the story of the dream that was more palatable for him to tell? Rather than confronting him with my suspicions, I preferred to engage him. "You know sexually transmitted infections come from real life encounters, not from dreams". He wished to know how certain I was about that. Even one hundred percent certainty did not convince him. Only a negative HIV test would convince him. I straightaway agreed to do the test. I needed, however, to explain that there is a window period of several weeks, up to two months, between a real exposure to HIV and development of the specific antibodies to be detected for diagnosis of HIV. We would therefore do two tests, the first there and then and he could come to pick up the results after one week and if this test turned out to be negative as expected, he might want to return after two months and repeat the test. Amnon paled: two months until certainty? Once again I tried extensively to reassure him: dreams, sexual fantasies, nocturnal emissions and masturbation did not lead to disease and definitely not to HIV. Purposefully I had mentioned sexual daydreaming, nocturnal emissions and masturbation. I knew these naïve yeshiva boys and their "sins": the vast majority entered marriage without sexual experience. Upon my words he burst into tears. A marriage arrangement was imminent, with the angel-like daughter of a local rabbi, he had experienced nocturnal emissions and he felt awful and embarrassed that he might cause an infection in his new wife. I was glad to have more of the truth and we had an instructing talk about sexuality and marriage. I referred him to several books on the topic, including by religious authors. He appeared relieved when he left, or perhaps I hoped and needed he was so? I did not expect an invitation to his wedding and indeed did not receive one. He did not return after two months for retesting.

About one and a half years later I received a phone call from a local walk-in clinic. The doctor who called described the case at hand. He attended a young man with a urethral discharge, indicative of gonococcal urethritis or non-specific urethritis, both common sexually transmitted infections. The doctor, who had trained in emergency medicine in the US, had run a rapid plasma reagin (RPR) test, which was positive, indicating exposure to syphilis. The doctor was appropriately concerned that the presence of two concomitant STDs could be indicative of additional ones and wished to test for all contingencies. What should be tested and what treatment should be provided? We agreed on a urethral swab for Gram stain and culture to rule out gonorrhea; and a blood test for syphilis, HIV (the human immunodeficiency virus causing AIDS), herpes simplex and viral hepatitis B and C. The patient would receive one intramuscular injection of the antibiotic ceftriaxone to cure possible gonorrhea and one oral dose of another antibiotic, azithromycin to cure non-specific urethritis. The tests were sent to our hospital's clinical laboratory, as the walk-in clinic's lab did not perform more than the most basic tests. Would I be willing to see the patient for follow-up?

Next week in clinic I immediately recognized Amnon Davidson, if only because of my handwriting in the chart from his previous clinic visit. However, only after he handed me a bunch of lab results and the referral letter from the walk-in clinic did the connection dawn on to me. The lab results indicated a positive gonorrhea culture, the non-specific syphilis blood test was positive at a titration of 1: 32, a specific test for syphilis was positive and confirmed the non-specific test, while HIV and viral hepatitis B were negative. This time I knew there would be no talk about dreams: this time was for real. "So Amnon, please tell me how you are doing". He appeared much more mature, but shadows had appeared under his eyes. He was reluctant to start talking, he would need more reassurance. "Please Amnon, I am just as human as you. I am your doctor, not your judge. Even our greatest sages, such as Maimonides used to say that there is no righteous man on earth who does not make mistakes. Jews believe that we should confess our mistakes, repent ("tshuvah" in Hebrew, symbolically indicating a return to God) and return to our original and pure self. Moreover, we believe that once we have made successful repentance we are better and stronger than we were before that sin: it won't happen again". "Thank you", he said in a soft voice, "under these circumstances it is perhaps God's hand that directed me to you once again. Please tell me what to do". Because Amnon was evidently not yet going to unburden himself, I said we would start discussing the diagnoses of his sexually transmitted infections, the treatment plan, and finally we would discuss how to prevent this from occurring again. Amnon had two concurrent infections, of which one symptomatic, while the other was silent and potentially more serious. The gonococcal infection of the urethra led to painful urination and a pussy discharge, which had led him to seek medical attention. Gonococcal infection of the urethra is occasionally accompanied by a chlamydial infection and, therefore, he had received treatment for both infections at the walk-in clinic, which should have cured his urethritis. Amnon confirmed that urination had become normal and the discharge had disappeared within a day after receiving the antibiotics. "You said there was something else, silent, potentially more dangerous?" I was glad that he had said something: we were on track of a more normal, bilateral conversation. "Yes indeed, the other infection is syphilis". He had never heard of it. I was not surprised of that: syphilis has been rare in Israel since many decades and Amnon lived in a secluded yeshiva world. However, I was surprised to encounter a patient with a high titer RPR test, indicating a relatively recent exposure to syphilis. This disease usually starts with a painless genital ulcer that spontaneously heals within several weeks. Several weeks later, in some but not all patients a secondary stage may occur, with headache, a general rash and multiple combinations of symptoms involving various body systems and organs. Untreated, this phase too will subside, after which patients enter a long "latent" asymptomatic period which may remain asymptomatic for the duration of the patient's life. However, a significant percent of patients may develop devastating neurological and/or vascular manifestations. The general and medical literature is awash with stories of the terrible toll this disease has extracted from men, women and children since the early 16th century. Entire monarchies have come down due to syphilis and the course of European history has been altered because of it. I concluded with a simply stated question: "Amnon, do you recall having had a small lesion on your penis in the last year or so?"

He flushed. Yes, about two months ago he had had a small ulcer behind the head of his penis, in the groove indicating the ritual circumcision ever male Jew undergoes at eight-days of age. It had stayed for about three weeks and just by the time he wondered whether to see a doctor it had healed without scar. I told him that primary syphilis is quite rare in Israel, although in some countries entire epidemics rage. Therefore I wondered whether he had had sexual contact with a foreigner, male or female. Once again he flushed: "You are able to detect things I thought were hidden. However, even if you know this much, it is important for me that you know that I have never done an abomination with a man". I thanked Amnon for his trust and willingness to share delicate information, reiterated that I understood how difficult this was for him, but encouraged him to proceed.

It appeared that Amnon had suffered from sexual daydreaming and fantasies since his early adolescence. According to the best Jewish tradition, he had worked hard to conquer his "evil inclination", always tried to avert his eyes from women and read classic books on self discipline written by saintly men. He was fortunately bright and had been able to attend the best yeshivas, the last one of such quality that its boys were much sought after as potential husbands, while the bride's father often would support the young couple for several more years while the young husband pursued advanced studies. Amnon' sexual fantasies bothered him sufficiently that one day he consulted a teacher, wondering aloud whether he should get married, even if most of the boys in his yeshiva would not get married until two or three years later. This wise teacher did not need much information: vague, indirect talk was sufficient and he supported Amnon's quest. A suitable match was found and the marriage took place, about two months after he had come to my clinic for the first time. He felt very lucky with his new wife, Tamar, a very sweet and kind young woman from a very religious background, who worked as a kindergarten teacher, while he continued to study in a yeshiva for married men. The regularity of family life suited Amnon very well. He became more relaxed and was able to concentrate better on his studies and for more prolonged times. His wife's first two menstrual periods proved challenging for Amnon. With the onset of the menstrual period religious couples refrain from all physical contact for the duration of bleeding and an additional seven clean days, after which the woman submerges in a ritual bath and the couple renews intimacy. Fortunately, Tamar became quickly pregnant and everything was very well for them until the seventh month' of pregnancy when irregular spotting occurred, which lead to immediate physical separation between the couple, which continued until Tamar was delivered of a healthy girl, about three months ago.

Amnon interrupted the narrative to blow his nose. He was evidently reaching the crisis, the lowest point in his life, when it should have been a spiritual high with the birth of his first child. The regularity of family life had been marvelous, exactly as he had anticipated. However, after he had become used to its associated tranquility the complete and prolonged absence of physical contact quickly became unbearable. He became irritable, flooded with fantasies and felt terribly uncomfortable. Masturbation was out of the question: our arch father Jacob's grandson Onan had wasted his semen rather than have his wife become pregnant, which might detract from her beauty and he was punished with death. Amnon had heard that in the area of the old bus station in Tel Aviv many foreigner workers lived, among and with whom sexual permissiveness was common. One evening he took the bus to Tel Aviv and started walking around the dimly lit, dilapidated area. He was picked up by a foreign woman, maybe Thai and they had stayed at a hotel room or her department. Although he had given her money up front, only on the way home did he discover that his wallet had been emptied out. The penile ulcer appeared some ten days later.

During Amnon's discourse I had remained silent, with lowered head, only very briefly making eye content now and then to demonstrate my non-critical, but unabated attention. When he disclosed the presence of a genital ulcer several months earlier, it seemed that this was a simple case of early latent syphilis, defined by some but not all books as the asymptomatic but infectious period up to one year after a primary lesion. However, nothing is simple and definitely not with sexually transmitted diseases. The RPR titer of 1:32 was compatible with recent primary syphilis, although I had seen many cases with primary or recent syphilis with much higher titers, up to 1:1024 or higher. Over time the titers decrease, usually after a course of penicillin, but also untreated. Could and should I rely on the history of this "only one time slip"? Could this one encounter or an earlier one have occurred before his marriage? Primary, secondary and early latent syphilis are treated with one intramuscular injection with benzathine penicillin. Late latent is treated with three such doses, one week apart between the three injections. I decided on the latter option, perhaps excessive but it seemed in my patient's best interest. In addition, I had to take into account the possibility that his wife and baby had become infected. As these things crossed my mind, I planned the subsequent talk.

"Thank you, Amnon", I started "for telling all this to me. You know that confessing by itself is helpful, the first step on the path of healing, physically and emotionally". I explained that treatment for syphilis consists of three injections, of which he would receive the first one that day, while the second and third after exactly one and two weeks. That would lead to complete cure, to be confirmed by follow up blood tests over time. The tricky issue was that his wife and baby had to have the same RPR blood test to rule out syphilis. Did he want to take them to the family doctor with a referral letter, or would he rather take them to see me next week or the one after when he came for his second injection? Before leaving me, I would like to strengthen him with several ideas. First, I wished to draw his attention to a novel written by American author Irvin Yalom. In order to increase his attractiveness to Amnon, I mentioned that Yalom was Jewish, a fact which the author had divulged in another book, while I omitted that Yalom was a psychiatrist. "The Schopenhauer cure" concerned the story of a young man who suffered terribly from obsessive and compulsive sexual behavior. This book was very different from the religious literature yeshiva students are used to read. Nonetheless, the protagonist underwent a complete personal transformation and became cured of his sexual obsession in the process, indicating a first, perhaps lower step in a person's spiritual cure. Second, I told him of a famous rabbi, a Kabala scholar of wide renown, who several centuries ago had evidently suffered from sexual fantasies which almost entirely disrupted his concentration. Eventually his own rabbi advised him to take two years off and go abroad, in order to contemplate, speculate and meditate in seclusion and pray. This rabbi completely recovered from his affliction. Strikingly, he understood the vast importance of his problem, the struggle with his problem, and the associated personal transformation, which had been essential for his entire further development. In association with the issue at hand, I reminded him of the prophet Hosea in the bible. In vivid terms the prophet describes his suffering on account of his wife's transgressions, how she leaves him and goes after her lovers, to fall from bad to worse. All the while, Hosea continues to follow her and tries to take care of her at a distance and eventually rescues her out of the gutter, takes her into his home, not as his wife, but in order to have her confess, repent and entirely transform her life. Fascinatingly, Hosea grows to understand that his personal tragedy is a parable for the relationship between God and the Jewish people, who have forsaken their loving and caring Father to live frivolous lives of empty materialism and sensuality. Hosea, moreover, understands that God precisely has led him to meet this wife, in order that he, Hosea, will feel the tragedy of personal betrayal, which sets him on his life's destiny, to rebuke and teach the Jewish people. "Thank you", Amnon said quietly, and left.

He came by himself for his second injection. He appeared less flustered and apparently had done some soul searching. He had read "Schopenhauer," stories of Hassidism and had gone to pray at the cave of a famous Kabala sage near the city of Safed in the north of the country. He had decided he would bring his wife and child the next time he came, but he would like to plan together what we were going to tell his wife. "Amnon, *I* am not going to say anything to your wife because all this concerns *your* privacy. Only *you* are entitled to say anything about your medical condition and the possible implications for your family if you wish so". I was not going to let him off the hook easily. But I also hoped that he would use the momentum to grow personally by working through his conflict. "All right then", he had made up his mind. He thought he would tell his wife that he had had a medical problem in his past and with the doctor's help was on the way to complete cure without residual problems. A simple blood test would ascertain that his wife and baby were healthy and if God forbid otherwise, a simple antibiotic would take of the problem. In addition, he wanted to tell his wife that his medical problem had resulted from a conflict in his soul with which he had struggled several years. Only after getting it of his mind, sowing it into reality and staring into a horrendous abyss had he been able to conquer this evil inclination. Amnon knew that the struggle would continue, but he had recognized God's hand in the task he was given as well as His help to overcome the problem. His personal plight had the promise of becoming his great asset. He would assure Tamar that he loved her, that he was committed to her and their family's wellbeing and that he needed her as his helper for/against himself.

Amnon had accomplished an astounding amount of personal work within a mere week. The session with his wife transpired as Amnon had planned. Both she and the baby fortunately had negative syphilis tests. One year later Amnon returned to my clinic to repeat his RPR test, which had declined to 1:4 and most likely would become entirely negative within one or two more years. Only 23 years old, Amnon had become a more mature man. He now sported a full beard, his eyes were quiet and thoughtful and he expressed himself in slow, precise sentences. Although he had not officially changed from being Haredy, he divided his study time between Talmud and Hassidism. A new layer of Jewish studies had opened up, the inner meaning or soul of the Torah. No careless word would pass his lips: he now *knew* like Adam and Eve *knew* that what one sows in the world with talk and action also builds a world inside one's soul. Although still challenging, Amnon now cherished family purity, the twelve days of enforced physical separation starting with his wife's period. He now realized what a unique instrument the Torah had provided: to help man conquer his sexual instinct and help him direct its tremendous force for constructive purposes, to build and maintain his marital relationship and family, rather than let his sexual instinct take command and lead him down destructive alleys. During these twelve days of separation each of the couple of necessity retreats within, spends time and energy on their own growth and development. The joy of their subsequent meeting was boundless: they recognized their "old" spouse, but they were also thrilled to discover the refurbished, grown partner. He was grateful to God for giving him his predicament as well as the cure and appreciated that his doctor had been a faithful messenger in His hands. One day, he speculated, he would council yeshiva students on the afflictions of the body and the soul and how to handle these with honor. Maybe he would even write a book.

Chapter 9: Fever of unknown origin

Patients go to doctors for relief of suffering and hopeful attainment of cure. Accurate diagnosis is the essential first step before treatment can be prescribed that may be reasonably expected to lead to the desired outcome. Doctors make diagnoses by a complicated intellectual and intuitive process. They carefully listen to their patients' complaints and medical history and ask multiple questions to diagnose, or rule out various possibilities. The history is definitely the most important component of the diagnostic process for most if not all disease processes. A detailed physical examination and routine and targeted laboratory tests provide further data. Physicians in general and infectious disease specialists not less are anxious to make correct diagnoses, because the chance of cure increases with appropriate treatment and, vice versa, inappropriate treatment may lead to unnecessary complications. We also cherish the challenge and appreciate the satisfaction of a correct diagnosis that down the road leads to a patient's cure.

One medical entity that is initially often baffling concerns "fever of unknown origin" (FUO). Although febrile illnesses are extremely common, fever of unknown origin is not so common, because of its strict definition. Harrison's textbook of internal medicine defines four variants of FUO: first, classical FUO, initially defined in the 1970s refers to patients with fever of at least 38^0 C that lasts three weeks or more *and* at least a basic laboratory investigation has been performed. Second, there is FUO in hospitalized patients, which usually indicates a hospital-acquired complication. Third, FUO may occur in cancer patients who receive chemotherapy, as a result of which they have temporarily a very low white blood cell count, which exposes them to a host of infections. Finally, there is FUO in patients with the acquired immune-deficiency syndrome and as a consequence of a deteriorated immune system they tend to develop regular and opportunistic infections. The textbook lists hundreds of causes that may cause any of these four kinds of FUO. It is up to the physician to collect information from the history, physical examination and various tests, and analyze the data in order to reach one plausible diagnosis that explains all findings. Over my career I have seen several hundred patients with classical fever of unknown origin: some were easy to solve, others were surprising, while an occasional case proved extremely taxing. Such was the case of Jacob Lux.

Mr. Lux had come to the emergency department after referral by his family physician. He was a 60 year old lawyer, married and father of three children. He was usually healthy except for high blood pressure, which had been diagnosed some ten years earlier and had been under excellent control with three anti-hypertensive medications. Four days before onset of his fever he had returned from a ten day trip to Europe made together with his youngest son on the occasion of the son's Bar Mitsvah. It had not been an organized tour, as many families like to take. They had made their own plans and visited Paris, London and Holland, mainly Amsterdam and its surrounding countryside and villages. They had stayed at quality hotels. Although most of their meals had been had in restaurants, they also picnicked in woodlands and near lakes, but they had not been swimming. Two days after returning Mr. Lux developed diarrhea, consisting of three or four loose stools each day, without nausea or vomiting, with loss of appetite. Over the next two days these symptoms improved, but fever appeared, usually up to 38^0 C in the morning and intermittently climbing to 39^0 C in the evenings. There were no additional complaints. He went about his usual business for the first few days, but after one week of fever he went to see his family practitioner. According to Mr. Lux, his doctor examined him carefully and sent routine blood tests, including a complete blood count and differential, and blood chemistries. Most of the test results turned out to be non-informative, i.e. normal except for the sedimentation rate which at 70 mm/hour was moderately elevated. An increased sedimentation rates is a very sensitive indicator of an inflammatory process anywhere in the body, but it is non-specific: many illnesses may cause an elevation in sedimentation rate, C reactive protein and fibrinogen, together tellingly called non-specific markers of inflammation. When fever continued, a chest radiogram and abdominal ultrasound were performed, but both were normal. During the second week with fever his doctor had prescribed an oral penicillin antibiotic, but several days of taking this medication did not make any change. By now he had lost two kilograms in weight and his doctor referred him to the emergency department.

When I was called to see the patient - for a third opinion - he had been in hospital for several days, had undergone a battery of tests and had also been seen by another infectious disease consultant. We teach medical students and residents to approach FUO in a systematic fashion. Rather than consider separately various individual illnesses, one should address several main categories such as: first, infectious diseases; second, connective tissue disorders (such as lupus and rheumatoid arthritis) and vascular inflammatory conditions (i.e. vasculites); third, tumors; fourth, granulomatous diseases (including inflammatory bowel disease); and finally, miscellaneous conditions. Each of these five entities should then be individually opened up to consider a variety of illnesses to produce a differential diagnosis, i.e., a list of conditions that should fit the patient's symptoms, physical findings and laboratory and imaging results. The category of infectious diseases accounts for the most significant percentage of patients with classical FUO, up to about a quarter of all cases according to most modern case series of FUO. Most infectious diseases are diagnosed within less than the three week case limit that helps define FUO. As Mr. Lux's symptoms were of such sudden onset, without significant medical background and appearing directly after recent travel an infectious disease seemed the most likely cause. His attending physician and the infectious disease consultant had considered an entire range of infectious diseases and had sent many blood, urine, stool and serological tests to exclude these illnesses. Thick and thin blood smears were ordered to rule out parasitic illnesses, including Borrelia and malaria. Although the patient never had travelled to a malaria-infected country, airport malaria has been described: a mosquito bite could potentially transfer malaria from a traveling carrier of this infection to another traveler. Various viral infections such as cytomegalovirus and Epstein Barr virus were ruled out, as the patient had antibodies to these viruses indicating past exposure. Rickettsial infections were excluded with repeat serological tests, as were syphilis and the acquired immunodeficiency syndrome. Repeat blood cultures were sterile, which was not entirely reassuring because the patient had received oral penicillin prior to admission, which may notoriously interfere with blood cultures. A trans-esophageal echocardiogram was performed and confirmed entirely normal heart valves, virtually excluding endocarditis, a relatively rare infection of the heart valves – but a common cause of FUO. A CT scan was done of the head, chest and abdomen; the interpreting radiologist ruled out presence of any local abnormality, from abscesses to tumors. A spinal tap was done to obtain cerebrospinal fluid and various tests of this fluid ruled out presence of any problem. A bone marrow tap was obtained for culture and pathology and was entirely normal.

When I met Mr. Lux for the first time he looked quite ill, pale and depressed. He appeared a serious, reserved, but respectful person. He expressed full confidence in the hospital and its team and our ability to diagnose his problem and help him solve it – even if these goals so far had proven elusive. Carefully I went over the medical history, asking multiple questions regarding the recent trip to Europe and other travels, the well being of his son and other family members (all were well), possible exposure to pets (there were none), hobbies, medications, as well as possible other symptoms, including the most subtle ones. I carefully examined him, but not unexpectedly did not detect any abnormality as he had already been examined by several physicians and no pathological finding had been described. I reviewed all tests and imaging procedures, but nothing new came up. This patient had suffered from FUO for more than three weeks, his fever continued unabatedly and in spite of extensive investigation the diagnosis remained mysterious. At this point I was inclined, albeit reluctantly to broaden the differential diagnoses to include other conditions such as connective disease diseases (such as sero-negative rheumatoid arthritis and vasculitides), granulomatous diseases such as inflammatory bowel disease and other rare conditions. Blood tests for connective tissue disorders came back subsequently and were all negative and so was a complete digestive tract work-up. According to some case series of FUO, in up to a quarter of patients no definite diagnosis is made; fortunately, it seems that almost all of these patients attain spontaneous cure.

Over the next several days, Mr. Lux's case continued to hold my attention. I entered internet programs such as GIDEON and other search engines, combed through the literature of FUO and hoped for some "lightening" insight during one sleepless night. Doctors are not natural friends of lawyers, so we definitely did not want to miss the chance to diagnose the source of this patient's FUO and treat him accordingly. In frustrating cases such as these, I often go back to the patient and start from the beginning. However, rather than limiting myself to the medical history I ask the patient to tell me about himself, his background, family and career. I commit myself to being open-minded and open-hearted in order to pick up nuances, a dissonant of any kind, anything colorful or special in the course of the individual's life – and place his current illness in the timeframe of his life. In particular, I try to discern a possible symbolic association with his symptoms, but as may be expected this is often quite difficult. It appeared Mr. Lux had had a stable youth in a well-to-do neighborhood in Tel Aviv. His grandparents had fled from Germany after Hitler became chancellor in 1933 and his father, teenager at the time, grew up in mandate Palestine. His grandfather had been a physician and superb role model as gentleman-professional to Mr. Lux himself. His father had been a career officer after having served as heroic fighter in the underground during the turbulent years preceding Israeli independence. His mother's parents were immigrants from Casablanca in Morocco where her father had been a rich merchant. The family's home had always been a center of Jewish study and social life. Mr. Lux's wife Suzanne had attended a prestigious art school in France before the family moved to Israel. She was seven years younger than him. Like many Israeli couples, Mr. Lux met his wife in the army, while he was on reserve duty and she in regular service and they married soon after her discharge. During his twenties Mr. Lux studied law and his specialty became corporate law; he smiled briefly as if to dismiss any possible concerns I might have about him being a malpractice lawyer. He also studied business administration and had an MBA. During the next twenty years he served on the executive board of several large companies. Around the age of fifty he developed severe headaches, which he initially ascribed to job-related stress. When he was diagnosed with high blood pressure he underwent extensive testing but no underlying reason had been diagnosed. With several medications his blood pressure became normal and his headaches disappeared. Nonetheless, he decided to resign from his job: although he originally had loved the power-wielding and can-do management of large companies he felt burnt-out. He subsequently set up his own law-office, providing business and legal advice to small businesses. He felt there was some idealism in supporting these enterprises, which owners were often innovative, enthusiastic and hard-working, but poorly equipped to deal with the requirements of modern business. He usually spent at least an hour or two on the road each day commuting to his office and visiting his clients, but in the last year or so he felt tired of it and burnt-out. Therefore, some five months ago he had decided to start working from the family home. He lived in a spacious cottage and he had set aside two rooms for his office. He smiled a wry smile: "rather than travel to my office, my clients come to visit me".

Please tell me about your family, I asked. He smiled, obviously proud: "My wife is a real artist". He described the nice attic studio that he had built for her in their home, where she creates the most beautiful painted glass objects, from windowpanes for synagogues and hotels to cabinets and lanterns. In the last few years, with the children growing independent she has also had exhibitions at art galleries, locally and in various cities abroad. They had three children: their oldest son was twenty-eight years old, still single, and had studied medicine. He was currently doing a residency in hematology in a hospital in Tel Aviv. I already knew: this son had called me several times to inquire after his father and make suggestions regarding the work-up. I appreciated his pleasant voice, polite inquiries and total absence of criticism. Mr. Lux mentioned how proud he was of his son, who had become a "real caring doctor" like his own grandfather. Their daughter was 25, married and had a one year old baby boy. She and her husband both studied psychology. Mr. Lux smiled, this time a more joyful smile: he obviously loved the couple and his grandson. Finally, he said and once again an almost apologetic smile lit up his otherwise drawn and serious face, they had their 13 old Benyamin. The two of them had had a great time just planning their recent trip, although the actual execution had turned out even better. They had talked about many things, starting with the history of the family and that of their native country, to relations between men and women, politics and ideology.

Could I detect any lead in this ostentatiously completely normal story? I made a brief note of some major features in my patient's story. First, his ancestors fled from Nazi Germany, but before the war and I had not noticed any major trauma associated with that. Second, his father had been a decorated freedom fighter and officer, but Mr. Lux had not expressed even a shadow of inferiority feelings. Third, there had been a significant midlife career change, evidently because of high blood pressure, but, importantly, the patient himself had mentioned job-related stress and burn-out. The latter word had again appeared, when Mr. Lux described the recent move of his office to his home – and both times it had been expressed with obvious emotion. Fourth, he provided a description of harmonious family life. Although his wife hailed from Morocco, a very different background than his own Ashkenazi (European) one, they had much in common, such as a modern, humanistic and professional outlook. Nonetheless, I had met his elegant wife once or twice during my visits with the patient; although she expressed concern, I sensed the presence of tension between the couple, which I could not pinpoint any further. None of these issues provided the longed-for breakthrough insight.

While we were discussing Mr. Lux's case in various staff meetings, he was sent home for a vacation of several days. He came back on the appointed day obviously suffering from a headache. The attending physician on the medical floor where he was hospitalized, questioned him regarding headaches. It appeared that he had not suffered from headaches since he started anti-hypertensive medications some ten years earlier. However, in the last three or four months he had experienced headaches at least once a week or so, usually lasting a few hours and "nothing way as bad" as when his hypertension was diagnosed. His family physician had measured his blood pressure several times and that was under control. Did Mr. Lux suffer from neck pain or shoulder aches? Any joint or muscle pains? These questions had been asked multiple times and the patient had denied their presence; but he also had denied existence of headaches. The attending raised a new diagnostic possibility: temporal arteritis, an inflammatory process of large arteries, mainly involving the temporal arteries, which can usually be palpated bilaterally on the sides of the forehead. Although described in patients of Mr. Lux's age, this condition of unknown source generally occurs in elderly people and even then is a relatively rare disease. Temporal arteritis is generally accompanied by neck and shoulder aches and its onset is gradual over several months. Untreated it may lead to blindness secondary to involvement of the retinal arteries. An ultrasound examination of the arteries demonstrated the tale-telling halo sign and a bilateral full-length biopsy was obtained, which confirmed the diagnosis. Mr. Lux received a detailed explanation and was started on a large dose of prednisone, which would be tapered down over the next few months or year. The decreasing sedimentation rate often serves as guide for reducing the dose of prednisone until the patient attains complete cure. Almost all patients are completely cured within two years. Within forty eight hours of starting prednisone, Mr. Lux's fever had disappeared and he felt well. His appetite returned, his mood improved and newly found energy invigorated him. He was discharged for rheumatology clinic follow-up, obviously in great spirits and appreciative of the care he had received.

This was clearly the successful end of a challenging story. Or was it? In a quiet moment I reread the summary notes I had made after Mr. Lux recounted his personal life. I wondered whether he had moved his office to his home *because* of the onset of symptoms associated with temporal arteritis, however subtle these might have been. Possibly the described burn-out had precipitated that shift – and he developed temporal arteritis *after* the change, with or without association between this move and the disease. I had nothing specific to go after, only my intuition telling that two things did not fit: first, the expression "burn-out" had been emotionally expressed on two different occasions referring to two events many years apart. The second point was even fuzzier: perhaps there was some tension between my patient and his wife, but marital tensions are - at least intermittently - the rule rather than exception. Were these sufficient reasons to call Mr. Lux? Although not in medical malpractice, he was after all a lawyer. I did not want to expose myself to ridicule, talking with him about vague feelings regarding burn-out and his marriage and a possible, but unsubstantiated association between personal issues and the onset of vasculitis. After deliberating for several days, I decided to call. I was actually relieved that no one answered and I could leave a message, expressing my concern regarding his further well-being and wishing him a speedy and complete cure. When he did not return my call within the next week or so I felt I had done my duty: we had provided state-of-the-art medical care of our patient's medical problem and I also had attempted – albeit weakly - to discuss an emotional and perhaps social issue that most likely was not related to his medical problem.

Three weeks later Mr. Lux called. Did I remember him? He appreciated my phone call, he apologized for not getting back to me sooner, but he had been abroad with a client on a business trip. Although he had been scheduled to come to the rheumatology out-patient clinic as temporal arteritis is within the field of expertise of rheumatologists, he would like to come and see me too. Would that be possible?

When Mr. Lux came to my office he exuded confidence, vigor and well-being. He felt more energetic than in quite some time and was able to work and be busy for many hours on stretch. His mood was excellent, his appetite was superb and he had regained the lost weight. So, I asked innocently, what was the reason he wished to come and see me. It appeared his son, the resident in hematology, had extensively questioned his father regarding his hospital stay. He had read about his father's disease in the textbooks and internet and knew what he felt he needed to know as a physician-son regarding his father's disease. However, it appeared the son had been very interested in the process of hospitalization: how various doctors had interviewed his father; the cascade of investigations that had been done and whether his father had been informed and prepared; and how relations had been in-between the staff's members and with Mr. Lux in particular. Finally, and this appeared to be most intriguing to the young Dr. Lux, he had been deeply impressed that someone had actually interviewed his father regarding his life's story and major experiences. According to Mr. Lux his son had decided on hematology (blood diseases) as career choice because it would allow for long-term and very personal contact with his patients, who were often engaged in the struggle for their very existence and hence they were more inclined to be open-hearted and willing to share. Dr. Lux had convinced his father that the interview I had dedicated to listen to his life story had been exceptional and should be appreciated. As a result Mr. Lux himself had written an account of his life, similar to what he had told me but in greater detail. He wished to know whether this interview had made a contribution to my understanding of his case.

Quietly I deliberated for some moments. A virtual flood of ideas and feelings passed through in a mere few seconds. I have been aware since my student years that physicians and their patients are partners in a mutually beneficial relationship. Most physicians and especially those who do not engage in critical self observance are probably unaware of this. Many may actually feel professional paternalism towards their patients, although expression of such attitude is politically incorrect in the current age. In am convinced that *all* relations with *all* people, not excluding patients, provide important messages and feedback for personal development. We can and should learn from each of life's encounters and occurrences. Having said all this, the physician should keep in mind that his foremost responsibility concerns his patient's interest and wellbeing. I shared these thoughts with Mr. Lux – and he appreciated my honesty. I confirmed that I had obtained two insights from the story of his life as he had reviewed it: one more distinct and one vague insight, which in retrospect could shed some light on the onset and development of his physical illness. However, all this was entirely speculative and there was no proof whatsoever to relate between these issues. It was, therefore, not my intent to convince him of such an association; rather, upon his request and with due modesty, I would share my observations and if that was beneficial so the better, and if not, please just forget it all.

Mr. Lux was relaxed but eager. I told him how I had been struck with his twice using the word burn-out and with obvious emotion, describing job related issues some ten years apart. He had been aware of it and had given it some thought too. I asked him to quickly give some synonyms and associations with burn-out. He briefly closed then opened his eyes and reeled off: fire, more fire, burning bush, burning forest, air plane crash, twin tower attack, cigarette smoke, cancer. I thanked him for his cooperation. Could he possible associate between fire and temporal arteritis, in essence an inflammation of the arteries? His shook his head in surprise and said softly: "incredible, incredible". He realized that even the word inflammation includes the essence of fire. His arteries had been on fire. But how could we relate between the burn-out in his job and the fire in his arteries? Moreover, many people experience burn-out and do not develop inflammation of their arteries. These were excellent questions and we could continue speculating, without getting definite answers. I would confine myself to making two observations: first, it seemed that a similar trigger could lead to various symptoms and diseases in different people. This concept was well known in modern medicine, which recognizes psychosomatic disorders, conditions, in which a psychological source evidently precipitates or exacerbates totally different syndromes such as irritable bowel syndrome, duodenal ulcer, asthma or psoriasis. Chinese medicine views shingles involving the left or right side of the chest wall as two totally different diseases, although western medicine considers both as caused by the Herpes zoster virus and treats these identically. I assured him that even formulating good questions is challenging and may be a giant step towards gaining insight in one's life and diseases.

Mr. Lux did not look too convinced, although he had savored the theme of fire, i.e. job-associated burn-out and "burning" arteries. He would speculate about it. Before taking his leave, he wondered about the second insight I may have had - the vaguer one, he recalled - when he recounted his life's story. I squirmed in my chair, even more discomfort-able than when discussing my first insight. I wondered: was this discussion in my patient's best interest? Or was I pursuing my personal interest in possible associations between emotional and social problems, and physical illness? I did not know the answer to my dilemma. I only knew my patient had not forgotten the second point: if he had wished, consciously or not, he could have left it at that. I had to trust my intuition and hope for the best.

After collecting my thoughts, I mentioned I had been somewhat surprised about a certain contrast. On the one hand, he had described his family with enthusiasm and pride. On the other hand, however, I had noticed a certain tension between him and his wife during the two times I had seen them together. I apologized: it had been tangible, but I could not describe it any further. "Please tell me I am wrong and to back off". He frowned, his face a closed book. He remained silent for at least a minute or two, a long time in such a situation. I felt I had blown it. This intrusion in a personal matter probably frittered away the small gain and goodwill of the fire symbolism. Possibly he was considering the names of colleagues who would assist him to sue me? Finally he opened up. "Once again you have hit something straight on the head," he started and indeed, "there may be a real association with fire". It appeared he and Suzanne had always had a very close relationship. There were very different but appeared to complement each other. He was very male, rational and articulate, while Suzanne was very feminine, sentimental and artistic. They greatly appreciate each other's uniqueness and realized the benefits of their association. They had only experienced minor and never major marital discordance. However, in the last four-five months Suzanne appeared increasingly irritable. She would snap at him at tiny issues that never had been a problem. She would complain of inability to concentrate and her artistic work did not pan out as she wished. He actually ascribed this irritability to the onset of menopause. He had read in Wikipedia that the associated hormonal changes cause hot flashes and emotional instability and just waited for these clouds to dissipate.

Food for thought indeed! I chose to proceed in a circumspect way. Have you heard, I asked Mr. Lux, about the famous sage Rabbi Ishmael, who two millennia ago formulated the thirteen rules with which the entire Torah can be analyzed and studied? He had not: he was secular and had been to a synagogue only on the occasions of his own Bar Mitswah and his sons'. I would explain, to help him understand my association. One of R. Ishmael's thirteen rules states that issues that were ostentatiously totally different, but that shared certain core words should be studied for likely association. This came to my mind when he mentioned that his wife's irritability had started in the last four-five months. Quite possibly this was related to her menopause. However, the same time frame had been mentioned in another context: did he remember? Once again Mr. Lux remained silent for a minute or two, evidently submerged in thought. This time I was less anxious myself: I sensed we were onto something. You are right, he said: this is the same period since I moved my office to our home. And come to think of it, his wife *had* been reluctant when he raised the possibility of the move. She had made some reservations, but all had been irrational and vague and he had convinced her that he himself would be more relaxed and less energy depleted. He actually liked it a lot: he did his job, saw his wife much more during the day than ever and he appreciated the many small, daily interactions. Suzanne, on the other hand, appeared to avoid him. She was busy with household chores, on the phone with friends, or went out for meetings. It puzzled him, but he was not unduly worried; he knew that women's hormones may play roller coaster with their moods and expected things to clear up soon.

However, I would not let Mr. Lux get off the hook so easily. Did your wife's menopause start in the last few months, I asked. Menstrual irregularities and hot flashes had started a year or two ago, so there was no clear relationship. What if indeed his daily presence at home did disconcert Suzanne and had upset her own precious balance? He enjoyed seeing his wife multiple times each day; his wife evidently loved him and their relationship and family, but this did not necessarily mean she needed or wished to meet that much. After all, throughout their marriage Mr. Lux had left home for work in the morning and returned in the evening, like in most families, while his wife's center had been at home, like in the traditional family of old. Even if nowadays many women leave home for work, Suzanne had made the family home her place of work, her castle. Her husband had changed the balance radically. He made the connection almost seamlessly: "Maybe I have indeed set off a fire." After a moment he admitted: "You know, I have noticed that my occasional headaches of the last few months were mostly precipitated by Suzanne being particularly short-tempered at me, which is maybe also the reason I never volunteered the information." Something else dawned: "You know, my last name means light. I have never thought about the continuum between light and fire. It reminds me of a probably untrue story about how Archimedes focused sun light through a magnifying glass to set Roman warships on fire. In temperate concentrations light is a blessing, while at higher concentration it may become fire and burn everything in its wake. Perhaps the same is true for relationships?"

Silently we considered the symbolism of the situation. I suggested we terminate our meeting, not before suggesting that he could call me if he wished to meet again. In addition, I wished to suggest two books, which might provide some further depth into the issues we had raised. Although there are many books about relationships, Dr. Barbara DeAngeles has addressed aspects in her book "What women want men to know" that seemed particularly pertinent to Mr. Lux's case. She described in detail the emotional dependence of women on their men, which she ascribed in terms of evolution. From prehistoric times until quite recently, women were economically totally dependent on their husbands. In order to raise a family, they had to attract a man and keep him interested emotionally, physically and sexually. Their very life and existence would depend on that. According to DeAngeles, this message has been programmed into the very being of women up to the point that even today, when many women work and could be financially independent the subconscious program makes their thoughts and actions revolve around their husbands. The daytime presence of the husband at home, whereas he previously had been away at work, could quite well be very unsettling for his wife – as confirmed by numerous women in interviews and questionnaires. The second book was religiously oriented and therefore perhaps less accessible to Mr. Lux. I noticed I had pinched a sensitive nerve. The well-known Hassidic Rabbi Shalom Arush had dedicated one book "The garden of peace" to a detailed discussion and advice on how to attain and maintain peace at home. The author discussed at length the situation of the unemployed husband, who sleeps in and wanders around the home. This Rabbi, talking from much experience warns his male readers that their presence at home during the daytime is often upsetting for their wives and paralyzes their functioning. He also provided some deeper understanding into the male and especially female soul explaining their particular behavior and reactions – which we could discuss at some other time if he wished too, or he might perhaps wish to read the book?

Doctors occasionally receive small presents from their patients, personal signs of appreciation. Two years after the described meeting a messenger brought a large bouquet with beautiful flowers. When I opened the attached small envelope, I found the receipt of a donation that had been made to the hospital's research fund. In addition, there were two visiting cards of Mr. Lux: one card indicated that his business office was at his personal residence, while the other showed it to be in an office building down town. On the first card was handwritten "former", on the second card "latter". I was of course intrigued and called him on his office phone number. His secretary forwarded the call. "Thank you for calling", he said. He had felt uncomfortable to call by himself after so much time. However, for some time he had wanted to update me regarding certain developments, but somehow could not get himself to act. It had been his wife's initiative to send the flowers, and he had jumped on the opportunity. "Thank you for the flowers and donation. And I appreciate the unspoken message with the two cards. Please tell me about your health and well being". It appeared prednisone therapy had been tapered off and discontinued about six months earlier and there had been blissfully no sign of relapse of temporal arteritis up till the present. He had read the books I had recommended. As predicted, he had enjoyed the DeAngeles' book and it had opened the pathways to more books on the topic of marital relationships. Rabbi Arush's book had initially been more difficult to access, although he had forced himself to read it. Both books had convinced him regarding the difficulty his daytime presence at home might pose for his wife. One day, it had been Suzanne's birthday, he mentioned that he considered moving his business office somewhere else "in order to have a clean separation between work and home" – and he wondered how Suzanne felt about that. Her initial reaction had been one of anguish and she was genuinely concerned that there was something wrong with their relationship and perhaps he was moving out? He reassured her and that, on the opposite, he loved her very much and felt their relationship might benefit if he kept a clear distance between his work and family. He would not forget her subsequent reaction: she appeared genuinely relieved as if a huge burden had fallen off and started crying. He had rented an office in town, reduced his office hours and in the freed-up time took two university courses, one on Jewish thinking, the other on Jewish history. Several months into these courses he had reread R. Arush's book. This time he had been better able to appreciate the author's references to the very first chapter of the Bible and the spiritual interpretations pertaining to the deeper layers in the soul of men and women. Interestingly, in spite of his reduced workweek his income had increased. He smiled: he recalled one observation in the book that a person's income somehow depends on whether he honors his wife and meets her needs and those of his family.

Chapter 10: Leprosy: A case of drug toxicity only?

One day about ten years ago, I received an outside phone call, transferred by the hospital operator. The caller identified himself as Raúl Toledano; could I please spare him three minutes and listen to his story? It appeared that three years earlier he had received the diagnosis of leprosy and since then he was on double antibiotic treatment. Two weeks before his phone call he noticed that the white of his eyes were turning yellowish and his urine had turned dark. In his youth he had had viral hepatitis, which had started with similar symptoms although at that time he had also suffered from fever, which was not the case this time. He went to the emergency department of a local hospital, where some blood tests revealed he had hepatitis, but viral infection was ruled out. The doctors made the diagnosis of toxic hepatitis and ascribed it to rifampicin, one of the antibiotics he was taking. He was recommended to discontinue this drug, but after some deliberation among the doctors they suggested he continue with dapsone, the other antibiotic he received. After discharge from the hospital he saw the dermatologist who had made the initial diagnosis of leprosy and whom he had seen since then about once a year. She recommended that Raúl discontinue dapsone as well, obtain weekly blood tests until liver function tests had fully normalized and then resume dapsone. Would I please see him for a second opinion?

The specialty of infectious diseases covers many, many diseases. Textbooks of internal medicine devote two or three times more pages to infectious diseases than to any other body organ or system, including heart diseases. Accordingly, infectious disease consultants often become sub-specialists of specific areas of interest, such as infections in immune-compromised patients, hospital acquired infections or AIDS. As a medical student in the 1970s I had seen some patients with Hansen's disease, the alternative name of leprosy, called after the physician who first discovered the causative organism in 1873, even before Koch detected Mycobacterium tuberculosis. Those patients lived in a local sanatorium, rather for social than medical reasons. Since then I had seen only one patient with leprosy, during my fellowship in the US. That involved an immigrant from India, who had been diagnosed with lepromatous leprosy and who had the characteristic symmetric nodules and raised plaques on his arms, earlobes and face, resulting in the diagnostic and disfiguring lion-like face. Although I had taken care of patients with rifampicin toxicity, all those involved patients with tuberculosis and of course I was familiar with the care of that disease, drug complications and second-line therapy. Leprosy was not within my field of expertise. I explained all this to Mr. Toledano and suggested that he look for an expert dermatologist for his second opinion. However, he was adamant to see me. He had consulted with a central and disinterested agency and they had referred him to me for two reasons: to discuss the management of toxic hepatitis and the possible meaning of his disease.

At the time, the symbolism and deeper significance of diseases had held my fascination for a number of years. However, I did not advertise my interest, only occasionally discussed these aspects in cases where I expected my patients might benefit. I was somewhat embarrassed that word of my unusual interest had leaked out and would have to face that. Possibly because of that embarrassment I agreed to see him and of course I was thrilled to discuss the possible meaning of leprosy with a patient. I undertook to review the relevant chapters in the standard textbooks of internal medicine and infectious diseases before the patient's scheduled visit. Regarding the symbolic meaning of leprosy I felt I needed far less preparation, although that initial optimism would be seriously challenged. After all, leprosy is the one disease that has been most extensively described in the Torah (Pentateuch), with several chapters devoted to it, which I had read and studied many times. Biblical commentators have usually ascribed this disease to slander, supporting their case with various stories appearing throughout the bible. The best course was definitely to stay open minded and stay tuned to the patient's story and needs.

According to the standard textbooks, leprosy is a chronic infectious disease caused by Mycobacterium leprae. Clinical manifestations are largely confined to the skin, peripheral nervous system, upper respiratory tract, eyes and testicles. The unique affinity of M. leprae for peripheral nerves and certain immunological reactions are the major cause of the leprosy's manifestations. The propensity of the disease, if untreated, to result in characteristic deformities and the recognition that the disease is communicable from person to person have resulted in profound social stigma in many cultures. Nowadays, with early diagnosis and appropriate treatment, patients can lead normal lives in the community and visible manifestations and deformities can largely be prevented. Leprosy is almost exclusively a disease of the developing world, affecting areas of Asia, Africa, Latin America (mainly Brazil), and the Pacific. In Brazil, the majority of cases occur in the Amazon basin. Globally, there are estimated to be eight million patients living with leprosy. Peak onset is in adolescence and young adulthood. The route of transmission remains uncertain and may be multiple, including nasal droplets, contact with infected soil and possibly even insects. The incubation period, from transmission to clinical manifestation varies between two and forty years, but is generally five to seven years. Leprosy presents as a spectrum of symptoms, ranging from tuberculoid to lepromatous forms, while in-between these extremes are borderline tuberculoid and borderline lepromatous leprosy. The less severe form is tuberculoid leprosy: symptoms consist of few hypo-pigmented macules or plaques that are sharply demarcated, insensitive to touch and devoid of normal skin components such as sweat glands and hair and thus are dry and scaly. Peripheral nerves of arms, hands, legs and feet are most commonly involved and asymmetrically with increased sensitivity and associated muscle damage. On the other hand, patients with lepromatous leprosy present with symmetrically distributed nodules, raised plaques and diffuse involvement of the skin, which, when on the face, results in the lion-like face previously mentioned. Nerve involvement tends to be symmetric and more damaging than in the tuberculoid form. These patients may also suffer from involvement of the upper respiratory tract, the anterior chamber of the eye and the testes. Peripheral nerve damage of the hands may lead to significant deformities and loss of feeling, leading to loss of digits. Involvement of the nose leads to chronic congestion, destruction of the nasal cartilage and deformity. The eyes may become ulcerated; leprosy remains a common cause of blindness in certain developing countries. The organism may invade the testicles; therefore, men with lepromatous leprosy may suffer from infertility due to decreased or complete absence of sperm production, and impotence. Leprosy is readily diagnosed by its appearance and confirmed by the characteristic skin biopsy. The three principal drugs that have been found effective are dapsone, clofazimine and rifampin, and various schedules have been published. In tuberculoid leprosy the treatment may consist of dapsone for five years or dapsone with rifampin for six months. For lepromatous leprosy, which usually involves many more bacteria and skin structure damage, treatment may consist of rifampin for three years with dapsone for life, or alternative protocols with varying degrees of duration. Mr. Toledano's reported use of rifampin and dapsone for three years suggested that he was diagnosed with lepromatous leprosy.

We met in the out-patient clinic. Mr. Toledano was 48 years old, married and had two sons, twelve and ten years old. He was an architect by profession and educational buildings were his specialty. Although he was born in Cairo, Egypt, his parents had fled to Brazil after the young officers' uprising which ousted king Farouk in the early 1950s. Raúl had grown up in Rio the Janeiro, a city with a gust of life which he adored. He and his wife had immigrated to Israel shortly after their marriage when he was 35 years old and both his sons were born in Israel. His wife was a nurse, six years his junior and she worked in a local hospital. Raúl himself was employed by a large architectural firm, where he worked on educational buildings. They had adjusted rather well to the new country, socially and financially. Adjusted so well, that his wife wished to become pregnant again and perhaps give birth to a baby girl. After several unsuccessful months they turned to a fertility clinic, where some tests indicated that his wife was alright, but he himself suffered from a paucity of sperm cells or hypospermia. When Raúl mentioned to their doctor that he had had some skin lesions on his scrotum for some time, he was referred to the hospital's dermatology clinic. The dermatologist extensively questioned him regarding his background and then asked him to undress completely. It appeared Raúl had multiple nodules on his legs, accompanied by dry, scaly skin and areas of decreased feeling, which had gradually started to appear around the time of his marriage. Both he and his wife had never given it much thought as they did not bother him. On examination, the dermatologist also felt the nodules on his scrotum and drew his attention to additional skin lesions, macules and plaques on his abdomen and forearms. She wished to know whether his libido was as usual and he needed to confess that in the last few years it was considerably less than in the past. He himself had ascribed it to approaching middle age. She asked his permission to take a small punch biopsy to confirm the diagnosis and two weeks later Raúl and his wife received the official diagnosis: borderline lepromatous leprosy. They had been flabbergasted. Although they were modern, non-biased professionals, leprosy still carries a significant social stigma. Raúl could not recall ever having been in contact with someone with leprosy. He read everything he could on the internet and completely agreed with his doctor that he had been very lucky that his face and peripheral nerves so far had been spared, although his testicles were probably involved. Since then he had taken oral dapsone and rifampin, while the intent had been to discontinue the latter after three years, depending on his clinical response and continue with dapsone for life. During the time of treatment, no new skin lesions had appeared, some had improved, but the sperm counts had not increased, nor had his libido. Accordingly, he had agreed with his dermatologist to add another two years with both medications and see. At that point in time the jaundice appeared, of which he had told me during his initial phone call and rifampin-related liver toxicity was diagnosed.

My patient looked well. Although he was 48 years old, he could have been years younger. His face was tanned, "due to frequent visits to construction sites". His full hair was brown without graying and although stocky he was not overweight. I carefully examined him, saw the tale telling signs of nodules, scaly dry skin, and various macules on his arms, legs and scrotal skin. He showed me pictures taken three years earlier, prior to treatment and he had definitely improved a lot. We reviewed his most recent blood tests and his liver enzymes had almost completely normalized. I told him that we treat patients with tuberculosis with four medications, of which three may cause liver toxicity, one of which is rifampin. Liver function disturbances are not unusual and we usually "treat through" without change in therapy unless liver function tests increase to more than four- or fivefold. In his case his liver function tests had gone up to more than fivefold and had been accompanied by jaundice and his doctors had appropriately discontinued rifampin. However, once his liver was back to normal one could carefully try to reinstitute the medication and follow with blood tests. Had Raúl abstained from alcohol during these years? Actually he had not, and coming to think of it, he might have had more than his one usual drink a day in the last several months. He could not blame his doctor: he had been recommended to quit alcohol consumption while taking rifampin.

Raúl repeated the two questions, which had brought him to see me. First, he wished to discuss the management of his toxic hepatitis and, secondly, the possible meaning of his disease. Once again I accentuated that he should seek advice from a prominent dermatologist with experience in the care of patients with leprosy. I mentioned that there were alternatives to rifampin, including clofazemine and ciprofloxaxin. Clofazemine is often unacceptable to patients because of the red-bluish black darkening of the skin which occurs in almost all patients, although it disappears over several months after discontinuation of the drug. But the foremost question was, whether he should receive another drug, in addition to dapsone and for what duration. The major indication in his case appeared to be the testicular involvement, resulting in reduced libido and low sperm counts - although his wife, by now 42, had resigned her dream of an additional child. I wondered whether he had looked in the internet for a suitable consulting dermatologist with much experience in leprosy, possibly in India or in his native Brazil. Was a trip to such a consultant beyond his budget? He smiled politely: he could definitely afford such a trip. The conclusion of this visit was that I would prepare a list of suitable internationally-based consultants, Raúl would ask his own dermatologist to whom of these he should refer and preferably his dermatologist should provide him with a summary of his medical condition to be sent by email to the selected dermatologist prior to his visit. He wondered about his second question? I smiled: "Please settle first the mundane and practical task at hand; and if you then are still interested we'll schedule a special visit."

Half a year later he called. He had gone back to Rio de Janeiro to visit his elderly parents. Both in Rio and Sao Paolo he had consulted with dermatologists with extensive experience in the care of leprosy. Their recommendation was unanimous: add ciprofloxacin to dapsone, citing two advantages. First, ciprofloxacin was probably effective in killing M. leprae organisms not less than rifampin, and secondly, it penetrated the male genital tract better than most other drugs and accordingly the chance of cure of his testicles was greater. Some of his skin lesions continued to improve, his liver function tests remained normal and he felt well. However, his libido was still very much diminished, which is what motivated him to call me and see whether we could be working on the second issue he had raised: the possible meaning of his disease. I warned him we would be entering deep water, uncharted territory and success was far from guaranteed, but if he consented with these provisions I was prepared to go ahead.

Once again I was impressed how well Raúl looked, younger than his age and relaxed, ostentatiously in direct contrast with the stigma-bearing skin disease he suffered from and the testicular dysfunction, which would seriously trouble most men. I mentioned these thoughts and his face immediately clouded. He himself had wondered about this too. He and his wife too wondered whether he suffered from some emotional blockage. Throughout all these years he went about as usual with his business, his family and his social activities. Once on the beach with his children, some girl had drawn attention to his skin lesions and an adult had told her that "that gentleman probably has psoriasis, a very common skin ailment". He immediately put the incident aside, but he knew it was "back there in his mind". He really would like to start considering the possible meaning and impact this disease had on his inner being. I deliberated where to start: either with a brief review of ancient Jewish sources on the spiritual significance of leprosy in order to stimulate Raúl's own imagination; or by having Raúl review his life story and see what emotionally charged issues would pop up and try to connect with these. My intuition told me to start with the first mode and continue with the second, and pray for Divine supervision.

"Mr. Toledano, ("please call me Raúl") I wonder whether you have read about leprosy in biblical stories". It appeared he had read some ancient Indian texts from the sixth century BC on leprosy as well as the biblical description of the disease. His main internet reading consisted of modern medical approaches to leprosy, especially after encouragement from his wife. However, he had not had that much of a Jewish education, so he had read the relevant biblical portions in French and Portuguese translation, and "many things get lost in translation". How come he knew French? It appeared Raúl's parents had spoken French in Egypt, like many citizens of European descent, Jews and gentile alike. His parents' ancestors originated from Toledo, Spain, where a very well educated Jewish community had thrived over several hundred years until the Iberian king Ferdinand had evicted all Jewry in 1492. The family name Toledano was reminiscent of that history. Raúl's great-grandfather, his father's grandfather had been a rabbi. The next generations had become secular and went into commerce due to a combination of factors such as European cultural influence and the economic conditions prevailing in Egypt. He felt himself a contradiction: in modern Israel Jews of Ashkenazi (European) descent were often either very religious or totally unobservant, while Jews of Sephardic (Spanish) background where almost all either religious or at least from traditional homes. Raúl himself was of Sephardic background, but his entire education had been like that of a Jew from any assimilated western European Ashkenazi setting. In Rio he had attended a regular elementary school, supplemented by some Jewish classes on Sundays. He remembered some very basic biblical stories, but once in junior high school he had rebelled and discontinued attendance. He remembered his father once or twice tried to reason him into re-enrolling. However, his mother, who hailed from an even more assimilated family, had supported him and he had appreciated her support. I was fascinated by his colorful history, while Raúl was evidently thrilled not less by the following brief review of leprosy in ancient Jewish literature.

Most biblical sources and commentators have ascribed leprosy to slander – and they have supported this contention with various biblical stories. The first story concerns Moses himself, who after being ordered by God to lead the Jewish people out of Egypt attempts to raise all kind of reasons why he should not assume this daunting task. One of his concerns was that the Jews would not believe him that he was ordered by God himself to lead them. This argument was countered by a sign: upon retrieving his hand from his cloak it was covered with leprosy, while reinserting it led to complete cure. While this sign ostentatiously would assist him convince possible doubters, it also served as a warning to Moses. He had slandered the Jewish people by suggesting they would not believe him, while in fact they did – and leprosy was the immediate punishment. A second story concerned his sister Miriam: her skin erupted with leprosy immediately after talking about her brother's abstinence from marital relations. Moses' prayer and one week of complete isolation led to cure. A third story concerns the prophet Elisha's aid Gihazy, who lied to a Syrian general after Elisha had cured him of leprosy by having him dip seven times in the Jordan river. The happy general wished to abundantly reward Elisha, but the prophet preferred to let him offer thankful prayers to God who had given the real cure. After taking his leave, the converted general went home. Unprompted, Gihazy went after the general and pretended in Elisha's name to obtain financial reward. The tit-for-tat result was leprosy, which affected Gihazy for his entire life. There are additional biblical stories that the sages quote to demonstrate that leprosy is indeed the result of slander, i.e. unsolicited talk about other people not present at the conversation.

Raúl raised several objections. First, although Miriam had talked about her brother the other two stories were not clear-cut cases of slander. Moses was legitimately concerned that the Jews might not accept his leadership; and Gihazy had lied for gain rather than slander Elisha. Second, he recalled that the biblical figure Joseph had actually informed on his brothers' misbehavior to their father Jacob, while the word slander was specifically used to describe that situation. Joseph never developed leprosy and for his haughty behavior regarding his brothers he had been sold into slavery, an entirely different punishment. Third, many people Raúl knew and perhaps all men, talk about other people. While in view of our conversation he was inclined to deplore this despicable habit, most gossipers evidently did and do get away unpunished. Finally and perhaps most important, what is the chain of events between a moral characteristic, i.e., slandering people that eventually leads to leprosy.

I was very much impressed with Raúl's objections and I commended him for not excepting my stories superficially. Indeed, if our discussion would lead to any productive insight, they would require his complete intellectual and emotional involvement. I engaged his arguments point by point. "Regarding your first objection, you are completely right. Biblical commentators have raised the same reservations. Perhaps their realization that the mentioned stories were not definite proof led to citation of multiple stories to bolster the case for a linkage. They also recited instances where people developed leprosy evidently as punishment for an entirely different offense. One such case involves king Uziah, some 700 BCE, who had the audacity to enter the holy Temple in Jerusalem and burn an incense offering, two actions that are restricted by law to priests only. When the high priest Azarya and other priests severely admonished him, Uziah became livid and turned around to vent his anger and everyone around including the king himself saw that leprosy had suddenly flourished on his forehead. Uziah remained a leper for life, involving loss of office and complete social seclusion, punishment for audacity rather than slander. Indeed, the sages list a number of other misbehaviors that might be punished by leprosy, as well as cases of slander that are punished otherwise, including that of Joseph and his brothers. Raúl's third point, that many obvious gossipers are not discernibly punished, raises the fascinating and disturbing issue of righteous persons, who suffer terrible adversity and that of overt criminals who seem to get away without punishment. Many key sages have thought about and discussed these issues in relevant treatises. As we were discussing a real person with leprosy I felt it was perhaps not really relevant to discuss inappropriate behavior that gets away unpunished, but rather focus on what might possibly be inner sources related to leprosy. Nonetheless, we would save the topic and perhaps discuss it at another time. His final point was definitely the most challenging: how could one explain the chain of events leading from a moral offense to a physical disease. Indeed, the ancient sources make only oblique reference to this issue. Modern medicine does not concern itself with the possible emotional or spiritual source of physical diseases. Most physicians would actually deny any causal relationship citing lack of demonstrable evidence. However, from an early age I have been fascinated by this question: because the single most vividly described illness in the bible, leprosy, is so distinctly ascribed to slander. The Hebrew words for slander and leprosy are intrinsically linked, which may suggest, but does not prove a causal relationship.

So, I suggested, let us consider the implications of slander. However, let me first take one step back: maybe we will be able to show a link between a moral offense and development of a physical illness. However, the mentioned biblical literature suggests that slander but other misbehavior too may lead to leprosy, while similar misconduct could also be unpunished. There is, therefore, much more to think about. Indeed, if anything, this discussion is meant to induce introspection and soul searching rather than provide clear-cut proof of a body-soul connection. I reassured Raúl that this discussion would definitely not incriminate him with some particular bad characteristic. Perhaps that would have been easier, because man prefers to cope with well described issues, even problematic ones rather than deal with uncertainty. Nonetheless, if anything, I would wish to set him on the unique path of self discovery with all its inherent uncertainty.

Raúl's face and body language indicated relief. I knew this talk must have taxed his emotional reserves considerably. However, he had requested the discussion; and moreover, building emotional suspense was probably necessary in order to have him fully engaged. "So", he said after relaxing somewhat, "what is your theory regarding the link between emotional issues and physical illness?" I admit: my appreciation for this intelligent and maturing person in front of me grew continuingly. "You are right: the signs are subtle and we are talking theory indeed. But modern medicine is very familiar with diseases of lifestyle. We know that smoking, obesity and lack of physical exercise are serious risk factors leading to diseases as diabetes, high blood pressure, heart disease, vascular blockages, stroke and even some forms of cancer. Then there is alcohol and drug abuse. Against their better judgment many people remain addicted to their unhealthy lifestyles. There must be some serious inner mechanisms that keep people locked into behavior that may lead to serious illness and shortened lifespan; and conversely, it takes considerable motivation to overcome those self destructive mechanisms. Many methods have been employed to increase a person's motivation to overcome their addiction to unhealthy lifestyle patterns, including behavioral techniques, social reinforcement, and emotional and spiritual methods. Now let us consider the common human trait of gossip". One famous sage, Rabbi Israel Meir of Radin wrote a famous treatise entitled Chafetz Chaim ("Lover of Life"), demonstrating the huge creative and, alternatively, destructive power of words. Nothing is as destructive as talk about other people. Rabbi Israel Meir provides a series of highly instructive teachings to employ only uncontaminated talk and avoid the seductive pit of slander. In fact, gossip erects walls between people instead of uniting people in a common brotherhood (see for example Beethoven's ninth symphony and Schiller's hymn concluding it, as well as numerous manifestations yearning for love and peace expressed over the ages in literature, art and even politics). These walls separate people. When someone gossips he actually judges the other person, who is usually absent and cannot defend himself, and ostentatiously places oneself above the other. Society fractures rather than unites. Leprosy consists of disfiguring skin lesions, leading to complete expulsion from society in the past and even to social isolation of the affected individual in the present. The sages recognized the symbolic nature of leprosy: the gossiper, who with his language ostracizes the victim of his words, becomes socially isolated as a result of leprosy. This is not proof of a chain of events, leading from slander to leprosy. It is a suggestion only. Down to earth realists may laugh at, or frown on this theory. More subtle people recognize the intricate relationship between, on the one hand, personal behavior and use of language and, on the other, social ills, marital discontent, emotional distress and finally illness. I concluded my mini-monologue by stressing once again that it was not my intent or belief that Raúl's leprosy resulted from him being a gossiper. Rather I wished to suggest that character traits and behavior could eventually lead to social, emotional and physical illness. According to ancient wisdom, Jewish and from most other civilizations, all men are born with deficiencies and man's main purpose in life may well be the amendment of these deficiencies. Rather than sitting in a cave for many years and correcting oneself through meditation or prayer, like the famous Rabbi Shimon Bar Yochai did some 1800 years ago, most people live and act in the world. We sow into the physical world, by expressing our inner world with words and deeds; and subsequently we reap the results of our talk and action. In fact, most people spend considerable amounts of emotional energy and thought on the digestion of their life's events with their friends or spouses or even therapists. Rather than blaming other people for certain setbacks and misfortunes, one could and should introspect and diagnose one's deficiencies and attempt to correct these.

Raúl smiled. I had evidently touched some inner cord. "From here onward", I encouraged him, "the journey becomes highly personal. This is uncharted territory and may be lonely and frightening. But it is ultimately the most rewarding journey one can make in life". After pondering quietly for a minute or so, he observed that "if I understand you correctly, you are not suggesting that I have leprosy as a result of an addiction to gossip. But rather that I should examine my life's events and try to discern symbolic threads that have unique meaning to me". I felt elated: this down to earth architect, who admitted to never having spent time on introspection or read a book on psychology or new-ageism had quickly grasped very unfamiliar concepts. He continued: "As a result of this new understanding I would like to spontaneously tell you - and have also myself listen - to some main features of my life". I smiled and encouraged him to proceed, although I cautioned him upfront that this journey quite likely would require other professional assistance, which we would consider towards the conclusion of his visit.

Raúl resumed: "I told you of my infancy in Egypt and my parents' move to Brazil when I was a toddler. My parents were immigrants in a strange land. They slowly learned Portuguese, continued to speak French at home and have retained their foreign accent up to the present. My father is very social, which is probably the key to his business success. He built a textile factory from scratch, has become quite wealthy and has become a philanthropist contributor to many worthwhile causes. Although he is a very likeable person, he exudes success and social power, which became a problem to me when I was a teenager and young adult. I felt I had to compete and felt inferior to his social and financial prowess. My mother remained at home and raised the kids, which includes me and my younger sister. She is much more reserved and rarely accompanies my father to social activities. I loved talking to her about everything. My sister has moved to Israel several years before I did, has married and lives a very stable life. I, on the other hand, became the recalcitrant teenager. I was an excellent student at high school, but I spent much time partying. To me, carnival time in Río was heaven on earth. I am easy going, probably inherited from my father. However, whereas my father is very conservative I am flamboyant." Raúl smiled a pleasure-tinged smile that transformed into ruefulness. "I loved the partying, the fun, the no-string attached promiscuity. I just adored girls and they adored me. There is no way I could recall how many nights I have slept around." The memories once again lit up his face in a sunny smile and once again it turned into something close to sorrow. "After I completed high school with the highest possible honors my father wished me to enter college, study business administration or law. However, I had met a beautiful girl from a very poor family, living in one of Río's extensive favelas or squatter neighborhoods. Santa Marta is an infamous, but colorful squatter community on a steep hill cascading down to the most beautiful beaches in the world. You cannot imagine the disorder: there are no streets, only alleys, winding down between huts and simple dwellings made of the most rudimentary materials. It is simply the antithesis of the rich and ordered houses and suburbs where I had lived my entire life. People are so much more authentic: to me they seemed exuberant with life, as opposed to the stuffed and stifled people I had grown up with".

Raúl's face clouded and he remained silent for several seconds, caught in memories and emotions. After collecting himself, he resumed: "I lived with Donna for two years. My father refused to give me an allowance if I did not study and right he was. So I worked in all kind of odd jobs, cleaning, selling, repairing cars and broken electric appliances, but mainly I loved helping people improve their homes. I learned

I have good hands and a good technical insight into the nature and use of various cheap and throwaway materials. I gained a reputation of reinforcing simple dwellings to better withstand rain and storms and improve insulation against the summer heat. Donna worked on a local market, selling vegetables. The romantic shine of the place slowly wore off as I realized the squalor of the lives of most of Donna Marta inhabitants. Their lives were short, nasty and brutal, to paraphrase a politician of the nineteenth century describing the people of London's poorer neighborhoods. I became close to many people and saw their endless financial trouble and their many poorly attended health problems. They lacked everything which I had always taken for granted, like clean drinking water, a bathroom, healthy food. At the time I started realizing this, the first cracks in our love affair occurred and over time we started quarreling too. Donna got pregnant when we were both twenty. One day, when she was some ten weeks pregnant she complained of sudden and severe stomach pains. These are not uncommon in Santa Marta, because of contaminated water and food, so people usually wait until everything settles by itself. However, during that evening she collapsed. I took her to a local hospital, a miserable affair by itself. She was found to be in shock, her blood pressure barely measurable and she was rushed to the operating room. I remember subsequent events as in a dream. An ashen faced surgeon came out to inform me that Donna had died, evidently of severe intra-abdominal hemorrhage due to a ruptured ectopic pregnancy in a fallopian tube. I don't remember the funeral; she was probably cremated. I do remember the incessant wailing of her mother and sisters over the next few days. I was simply in shock myself, totally unprepared to meet death so young and suddenly and so close at hand".

Raúl looked up. "I guess this is one major issue that I haven't completely digested. I literally tried to run away from it. I had very little belongings, packed everything in a backpack and during the next several months hiked my way up and west through Brazil into the Amazon basin". He paused. "Brazil is beautiful. Nature is, but people are too. I had plenty to think about, which I didn't, and rather looked forward to more adventure and more interactions. I stayed over in some villages for several months at a time, earned my stay and food by helping in agriculture, or, increasingly, by offering to improve the villagers' simple homes. I would not recall the names of quite some of these villages or the names of the people I stayed with or girls I slept with. In one village of Indians I stayed for at least a year. I lived with a local girl, worked with her on the family plot, went out hunting with the men and participated in their cultural life. Life was simple, we were part of nature. We slept on mats on the ground". Once again Raúl paused. "You will probably not believe the following. My girl became pregnant. However, I was not concerned, because in Brazil so many children are born out of marriage. When she went into labor I was sent out and the village midwife came to assist. When I returned in the evening I found her usual talkative family pale-faced and quiet, busy making funeral arrangements. The baby had been born with his buttocks up front; it got stuck and suffocated, while his mother had bled to death". Raúl blinked: these memories were obviously still very emotional even after twenty five years.

"Several weeks later I took my leave. I had more or less decided to visit my parents. Although I had informed my parents at the time I left Río, I had not been in touch them for the five years or so that I had been wandering. I actually yearned to see them and for the first time felt guilty towards them. When I called them, on my way back, my mother burst in tears from relief. Once home, my mother silently listened to my accounts, as she was used to throughout my youth, while my father simply embraced me and just said: I am proud of you, don't have any complaints. The next day I went to the local public library and asked the librarian for a popular book on building or architecture. She scrutinized my face, and then asked whether I knew Ayn Rand's "The Fountainhead". As I had never heard about this author I loaned the book and during the next several days read it from cover to cover. I had found my calling: building, architecture and I would specialize in educational buildings, having realized the hard way how crucial education is for the welfare of individuals and society. My father agreed to support me throughout college, if I was fully committed. I can briefly summarize the following years. I was 25 years old when I returned from my drifting. During the next five years I studied diligently; although I lived in a rented room near the campus I went to see my parents twice weekly. After completion of my studies I took a job in a local architecture firm to gain experience. My first hand familiarity with construction has given me an edge above most architects: I know how to use my hands, to employ materials and above all how to deal with the down-to-earth people who do the actual construction. I then took a year of and went to a college in Boston for sub-specialization. Two years after my return to Río I met my wife at a bachelor party. Until then, although a dedicated professional I continued to live a free life of promiscuity".

I winced: Although Raúl had expressed some pangs of consciousness regarding his parents after returning from the Amazon his fascinating account had been by and large devoid of introspection or emotions. This was the first time he called his free living habits promiscuity. It appeared Raúl dated his wife for several months until she completed her nursing studies and to his parents' delight they decided to marry. They even supported their decision to immigrate to Israel. Although this initially surprised him, Raúl felt that his parents probably thought they would meet their children and future grandchildren more often in Israel than if they stayed on in Brazil. His parents had made regular visits to Israel ever since his sister had moved there; his own immigration would only increase their frequency. He concluded his account by confessing that after his marriage occasionally, but "much less than in the past" he continued to have casual encounters with other women. His wording and facial expression suggested that this was indeed a confession. What in the past had seemed completely normal to him had recently become somewhat repugnant. Time was passing: we agreed to terminate the current session and meet again in two weeks, not before I expressed my sincere appreciation for his frank disclosures and Raúl thanked me for this unique meeting.

As usual, I made a brief summary of the visit in the clinic chart. A chronological list of the major lifetime events is usually easiest and in this case too. Finally, I wondered, what were the major themes of this person's life? First, there was the backdrop of immigrant parents and cultural alienation and the son's overcompensation and easy absorption into local cultural backgrounds. Second, there was the towering presence of the self-made businessman father and the son's obvious need to grow up and out of his father's shadow. Third, perhaps his womanizing was a slap in the face of his father's conservatism and simultaneously a demonstration of the son's own virility. Fourth, two young "wives" die on account of obstetric complications, a common albeit terrible feature of poverty in developing countries. Fifth, design of buildings and of educational structures in particular were Raúl's compensative response to life's miseries as experienced by him. Last but not least there was leprosy. The rational infectious disease doctor within guessed that this patient had probably been exposed to leprosy during his stay in the Amazon, or, less likely, sexually. But I wondered about the elusive "host factors", individual characteristics which ultimately determine whether a patient falls ill and how serious his disease turns out. How to make this puzzle fit?

Raúl entered my office for our third meeting with evident eagerness. I did not need to ask him any question or jumpstart him. He wished to commence with several remarks. First, the previous meeting had been hugely important for him, a virtual eye-opener, starting with my quotations from ancient Jewish sources regarding the possible symbolic meaning of diseases and ending with his recounting of his life's main events. However, it had set off a virtual deluge of emotions, which had upset his usual composure, caused nights of insomnia and let to vivid and violent dreams. I reassured him: the road to personal freedom of necessity is tough and passes through minefields. Those mines are not to be avoided at all cost, which is what people do intuitively during their entire lives. Rather, one has to detect those mines, learn their anatomy and defuse them. The first conscious encounter with those minefields may precipitate attacks of panic and anxiety. However, the knowledge that this is the only and infallible way to attaining personal freedom may provide the courage to persist. One may choose to close one's eyes to those personal minefields in the hope they will fade away. They won't: the number of mines as well as their individual destructive power will only increase over time. In fact, one mine, leprosy already had exploded.

Raúl agreed. In fact, he had made a short list of major features in his life and had started considering possible associations. One major eureka moment had happened during one fitful night. The concept of tit-for-tit punishment had struck him profoundly as demonstrated by my recounting of the biblical story of Gihazy. He could not but make the direct association between his sexual promiscuity and the development of leprosy, which in his case had mainly affected his testicular and sexual functioning. He believed that the root cause of his sexual exploits was an unconscious wish to show his father that he, Raúl was a real, strong man in his own right. He felt that his years on the road, starting in the Dona Marta favela in Río, up to his extended stay in an Indian village in the Amazon rain forest probably all were an extended teenage rebellion. Finally, he was somewhat proud of the fact that the subsequent years all stood in the light of construction: the actual construction of buildings and in particular those that facilitated education, but also socially, with a stable marriage and raising a family. It dumb-folded him that particularly in the latter, constructive phase of his life a mine had exploded in the form of leprosy. What did I make of that?

As almost always, I was enchanted by the quickness with which people, who have never been very inwardly oriented, are willing and able to observe their life's events and are able to assess important emotions – provided a major life changing event or illness has erupted. I expressed my appreciation for the considerable homework he had done as well as his frankness. Of course I would not know the answer to his excellent question, although the ancient Jewish sages observe that there is often a significant latency between offenses and subsequent results, both in the life of the individual and that of an entire community. The sages suggest that if the individual or nation amends their ways and correct their behavior the punitive result may never materialize. According to that view, the ultimate purpose of illnesses and the setbacks of life are to precipitate introspection and corrective thinking, verbal expression and behavior.

Raúl quickly caught on to my very subtle message. "You may be right" he said. Although after his marriage he had significantly reduced his womanizing, it was still present "in the shadows". He had given it some serious thought. It seemed to him that most young women he had met were as eager as young men to have sexual encounters. However, once relationships last a year or so, there appears to be a waning of interest on both sides, but especially in women. This reduced interest diminishes even further during pregnancy and especially after childbirth. Raúl had often felt offended when his wife rejected his advances. Later, when he read or heard colleagues joke about "not tonight, honey" he understood that this was a common phenomenon. The way he figured it out was that once a woman has attracted a man and has him committed to marriage, sex diminishes into a mere means (to keep her man interested and committed) rather than a purpose in itself. Accordingly, it was not surprising to Raúl that so many men turn to extra-marital affairs.

Many self-help book and guides on sexuality discuss these themes, and of course I supported Raúl's insights. I wished, however, to take his observations two steps further. We agreed that sexual relations were an important force to maintain a marriage. He observed quite correctly that the initial passions wane over time. Indeed, they spawned and reinforced other forces, such as nurturing and care, mutual commitment, selflessness and dedication, especially in face of adversity. Sexuality for uneducated men (this time Raúl winced) is release and fun, to be had at any time and any circumstance. For women sex is usually a much more complicated matter. Firstly, their monthly period is associated with pain and unpleasantness. Second, sexuality may and does lead to pregnancy and childbirth, indicating a life-defining change of much greater impact than for men. Not surprisingly, women are programmed to be much more cautious about it. I waited a few seconds to have him digest things. "And the second step?" he reminded me. I had not forgotten, appreciated his willingness to proceed. I told him I felt the second step to be much more important. I asked him whether he had heard about "the family purity ritual", laws observed by all religious and many secular Jewish couples. Vaguely, he said, something with immersion in a ritual bath, or so. According to the Halachah (Jewish Law), couples discontinue having marital relations and refrain from any physical contact from the day before the expected onset of the monthly period to seven days after its discontinuation, usually about eleven or twelve days. The woman subsequently immerses into a ritual bath of specified proportions, consisting of natural, un-pumped water. This ostentatiously artificial separation fuels mutual anticipation and attraction. However, there is much more to it. During the days of separation each of the couple is of necessity withdrawn inside his or her own individuality. Libido is transmuted into personal development and growth: emotional, psychological and spiritual. Marriage is an undulating meeting of two individuals, who come together and separate and come together and separate. They are not supposed to mesh. They are supposed to help each develop and mature, each according to his and her inner program, a program that no one knows up front but slowly discovers throughout one's lifetime.

Raúl's eyes shone, his face radiating innocence that made him look even more youthful than usual. He savored the expressed ideas, almost as if tasting them. He carefully looked for words before expressing himself. "Once again you have surprised me and most delicately by showing that even things as natural and ordinary as sex may and should have an emotional and spiritual over-layer, intricately bound up with it". I reinforced his new insight: everything, starting with the most down-to-earth issue has an inner symbolic force that only needs to be revealed. Ultimately life becomes significant to man only after exposing and connecting that inner essence with the outer, worldly shell.

My job was completed. I had taken care of the biological component of my patient's illness. I could perfectly have signed off there and then, which any peer review would have condoned. However, I had shown him an entirely new direction and purpose. From here onwards he would be the driver and active force exploring his own life in an entirely new light. Although it was tempting to continue to serve as longer term therapist I almost invariably refrain from doing so. The necessary commitment in time, emotional energy and perhaps required expertise are beyond my scope as busy hospital-based physician. I suggested to Raúl several directions and gave him names of dedicated professionals, who could further assist him develop insights and techniques and provide expert guidance on the newly found path - before striking it out on his own and with his wife as ultimate partner in life.

Chapter 11: Second generation syndrome

Moses P seemed to have it all. He was a successful middle-aged family physician, healthy, happily married, with grown children and grandchildren. Nonetheless, he often felt overworked, stressed out by "too many things to do" and fatigued. He felt obliged to continuously take on new duties, felt an almost obsessive need to assist people whenever they asked him and, being highly sensitive to his environment even tried to meet unstated needs which he seemed to sense or guess. On the one hand he had to answer this inner call to duty, craved the ensuing respect from his patients and fellow men; while on the other hand he never seemed to deserve a break and compulsively went from one task to the other. Simultaneous multitasking had become part of his life and while being busy with performing one or more duties, his mind was already restlessly occupied with the errands ahead.

I met Moses years ago and we have had many conversations ever since. Being a fellow physician, and not defining himself a patient, he preferred to talk as friends rather than coming to see me in my clinic. Through Moses, I met with the second generation syndrome, an elusive complex of variable symptoms that appears to affect a significant percentage of children of holocaust survivors.

Moses' parents were teenagers in France during the Holocaust. They were hidden by kind gentiles, who took serious risks to do so. Moses' youth, during the 1950's and 1960's, was cast under the shadow of the Second World War, although it took him much observation and introspection to recognize this elusive shadow and its implications. His father told him of his wartime experiences: how, as a young teenager he was torn away from his family, fleeing from one address to another; of midnight betrayal; of having to trust Gentile strangers who transferred him by bike from place to place; of cruel persons, who oppressed the Jews thrust into their power; and of a village of kind Catholic families, who all took in Jews and cared for them until the end of the war. Moses learned about thankfulness from his father, who throughout his life maintained contact with his rescuers and their descendants. Except for his father and his father's nuclear family all cousins, aunts, uncles, grandparents were wiped out in the death machine created by that most cultured of all European nations. His mother was less communicative about the war; she, her parents and siblings were hidden each at a single address in the Loraine countryside. Although some aunts and uncles, and many friends and acquaintances "did not return" from the war, it seemed that her story was not heroic at all, perhaps even banal, considering the boredom of being hidden in a tiny room, attic or cellar. His mother's silence regarding her war time experience helped Moses understand something crucial regarding the entire generation of Holocaust survivors. They did not want to talk about the war almost as if they were embarrassed. The real heroes were evidently those who had perished. What could the survivors talk about: about the inconvenience of living in a dark and tiny room, about perpetual hunger, the perpetual fear of betrayal? Perhaps there was a tinge of shame regarding those who did not survive, perhaps a sense of duty towards those to pick up things and make a new life.

Israel provided that new life. Many of the Holocaust survivors, especially the young, could not face life in the old country. They were forever asking themselves, how their neighbors, their customers, the people in the street had behaved towards the Jews. Had they been good Gentiles; or, like most, indifferent, perhaps unable to do anything to help; or, had they, like so many, been active collaborators with the Nazi's? Moses' parents, individually, left their respective families to immigrate to Israel, while their parents mourned their departure: still miserable after the loss of so many close ones, the departure of a child to a nascent country still in the throes of war itself, in an age with few modern means of communication or transportation, indicated a real loss. Moses was born in Israel in the early 1950's, but while still a toddler his parents returned to their native France due to various family reasons. They settled in the town of his mother's youth, an industrial town in the north-east of France: its Jewish community consisted of a handful of families, a pitiful remnant of the large community who had lived there before the war.

The shadow of the Holocaust was difficult to define and recognize. The damage the town had sustained by allied bombing and German misbehavior during the war had been entirely repaired. Society functioned perfectly. But the Jews were gone, save a handful of survivors, many ill or handicapped, and all emotionally traumatized. Moses' parents, although not religiously observant, were official members of the synagogue and the tiny remnant of the Jewish community, in order to maintain their Jewish identity and sent him to a religious youth movement for twice yearly meetings. Most of those who attended maintained their Jewish identity, many immigrated to Israel. With the Zionist education he received at home and in the youth movement, he left for Israel after completing high school.

During the subsequent decades Moses completely integrated into Israeli society, did army service, became a physician, married and raised a family. Nonetheless, the Holocaust continued to cast its shadow, which actually seemed to darken as time passed. With time and introspection he gained insight into his symptoms of obsessive compulsive activity, at the root of which he believed was the subconscious heavy responsibility to live for his murdered ancestors and the subconscious wish to give pride and joy to his war-scarred parents. He also understood that, paradoxically he had become attached or addicted to the depressive mood and mentality of being a second generation Holocaust survivor. The shadow of disaster and death seemed to provide a measure of meaning. With these personal insights, Moses also developed greater understanding regarding psycho-social trends in Israeli society.

During the first two decades after Independence very little public attention was paid to holocaust survivors. The real Israeli heroes were the soldiers who fought in the Israel Defense Forces; holocaust survivors were viewed with a mixture of pity and incredibility. How come they have led themselves being slaughtered like sheep? Only gradually, over the ensuing decades, has the Israeli public become better informed about life in the Diaspora up to and during the Nazi period. In the first two-three decades everything was about the New Society being built in Israel and little time or thought was spent on what happened before, either in the recent or remote past. Holocaust Remembrance Day fell very much in the shadow of the Day of Remembrance for the soldiers, who sacrificed their lives in the wars and actions for Israel's struggle for survival. However, in the last two decades the Holocaust and its survivors have gained a new honor and standing. The ceremonies of Holocaust day and their attendance do not fall below those of soldiers' Remembrance Day. The Yad Vashem Holocaust museum in Jerusalem has been totally renovated and draws large crowds from all sectors of society, including Sephardic Jews, hailing from countries, which Jews suffered various disasters but not Nazi occupation. High school children attend weeklong journeys to Poland and the death camps, after being prepared during the year prior to the trip.

It often seemed to Moses that the Holocaust had become a pseudo-religion or at least a state of mind. In the past only Holocaust survivors would point an accusing finger at the world, while it has become normative for all Israelis to do so. The Holocaust, representing the ultimate act of anti-Semitism in a many centuries' long chain of hostility towards Jews everywhere, seemingly has become the pseudo common religion, uniting the religious and secular, Ashkenazi and Sephardic, young and old, immigrants with the native born. However, it is a pseudo-religion, perhaps indicating the current state of cultural and spiritual development in Israel. The Holocaust is essentially the mass murder of European Jewry, the most efficiently organized pogrom carried out by western societies against their Jewish citizens. It is a history of and monument to Death. Judaism celebrates life, abhors death. The Bible and Talmud call death the ultimate father of impurity. Ancient Egypt celebrated death, with its pyramids, tombs and mummies of Pharaohs. Jewish religion has radically deviated from the ancient Egyptian culture. So how come that the Holocaust has become a pseudo-religion, uniting the opposing components of Israeli society?

The answer to that question seemed to Moses: it has filled a void created by two forces. First, although Israel's founding generations from the 1880s till the first world war, mostly hailed from religious families of eastern-European origin, they turned against their roots, to become modern, a-religious Zionists. They were rooted in Jewish thought and culture, although they turned the page on their background, identifying that background with failure and persecution. The next generation(s) grew up without much education in Judaism, but also without the anger of their parents against that background. Second and closely related, Zionism as ideology suffered the fate of its own success: Zionism as a political movement has succeeded as few political movements have. Israel has become a modern, developed country and Zionism as a political, idealistic movement has run out of steam. The Holocaust culture fills this gap in the hearts and minds of many Israelis. However, it is a pseudo-religion and serves for the moment, until the people and the country are ready to embark on the next step of emotional and spiritual development. How much easier to point an accusing finger at the Nazis, the Germans, the Christians, the Muslims, rather than look inward, to search our individual and collective souls.

According to the sages of the Talmud, the first Temple was destroyed on account of "idolatry, bloodshed and incest", while the second Temple was destroyed by "pointless dislike" among the Jews. However, history records that the first Temple was destroyed in 585 BC by Nebuchadnezzar, king of the Babylonians, while the second Temple was sacked by Titus and the Romans. The telling discrepancy between these radically different worldviews is also demonstrated in a well-known Midrash (legend) of two famous rabbis, rabbi Ishmael and rabbi Shimon ben Gamliel living during the Roman occupation and persecutions, some two thousand years ago.

The Roman ruler during their time had read in the Torah that stealing a fellow man and selling him into slavery carried the death penalty. Joseph's brothers, who had sold him into slavery, had got away with that sin; therefore, 10 sages would be killed to atone for that omission, along whom rabbi Ishmael and rabbi Shimon. On the way to their death rabbi Shimon asked rabbi Ishmael, what they had done that God brought on their death this way. Rabbi Ishmael mentioned that they may have let wait a widow or orphan coming for their legal assistance and the Torah is very strict about that, punishing misbehavior against the socially weak with death. Upon this explanation, Rabbi Shimon thanked his teacher "for this consoling explanation". To most of us, being led to such a "random" death for such a minor issue would generate feelings of intense anger, frustration and expressions of hatred against the barbarian oppressor. To these sages, their death evidently came from God and the Romans were just His unknowing instruments. Moreover, each event occurring in our lives should lead to introspection, verbal confession and rectification, a change in thinking, talking and behavior.

Twice in the Torah a long chapter is devoted to the punishments awaiting the Jewish people if and when they astray from the commandments. These chapters start out by describing the extensive blessings being bestowed upon the Jews by following God's commandments. Peace, health, fertility, plentitude of everything. However, God predicted to Moses before his death that the people would stop following His way and punishments would be severe, both for the individual and for the nation, including persecution and exile among the nations. The first version describes ever increasing severity of punishments until resistance to the Torah's commands are broken, loathing from the commands will turn into love, the people will return to God and His way and He will return the Jews to Israel. The second version just gives the list of punishments, twice as detailed at the earlier one, one uninterrupted flood of calamities. However, it ends with the same promise of redemption for the surviving remnant of Jewry, who will return to the Land of Promise and follow the Torah's commands and announce His Name and way to the nations.

Holocaust survivors, Jews and Israelis, religious and secular, are still very much in the phase of blaming the Nazis, the Germans and their collaborators and the world at large for all the persecution and horrors they have brought upon the Jews throughout the ages up till the present day. Yes indeed, all are guilty, either as active perpetrators or as passive bystanders. Even if they are unwitting instruments in the hands of God, that does not absolve the perpetrators of guilt and punishment. In the story of Joseph and his brothers, the Torah shows the ingenuous way by which the Divine plans are executed. God had announced a terrible prophesy to Abraham: that his descendants would become enslaved by a foreign nation. However, this would mold them into a nation and they would eventually be freed by His hand and return to the Land of Promise with great riches. Moreover, their oppressors would receive severe judgment, meticulously carried out according to the Book of Exodus. If the enslaving Egyptians were mere instruments in His hands, why should they deserve punishment? According to Jewish understanding, man has a free choice. Even if it is predicted that man will act in a certain evil way, he has a free choice, can and should introspect, change his innate inclinations, and think, talk and behave in a corrected, superior way: His way. The story of Joseph and his brothers makes this point in a most intricate, delicate and persuasive fashion. Joseph, the youngest of his family, is sold by his brothers into Egyptian slavery, their motive being hatred brought on by sibling rivalry. After thirteen years of suffering, introspection and internal growth, Joseph becomes viceroy of Egypt. Famine in Canaan leads his brothers to Egypt, where Joseph's wise and God inspired rule has lead to plenitude. The brothers, having had to witness their father Jacob's suffering during the two decades of Joseph's disappearance, are torn by remorse and regret. Joseph puts his brothers, who do not recognize him, through a chain of events that step by step leads them to complete repentance and a totally different mode of behavior. Jacob and the careful reader understand that the prophesy made to Abraham is carried out through the brothers' sale of Joseph. Nonetheless, that does not absolve the brothers of guilt and punishment. However, as is made abundantly clear, God does not seek punishment, as the barbarian Roman ruler thought, who executed ten wise men to make up for the sale by the ten brothers according to an infantile understanding of the "eye for an eye" rule. God has created man with all his inherent failings, to have him act and sow in the world, in order to gain insight in his own soul and gradually and continually improve himself. These are among the important messages of the biblical story of Joseph.

Moses' insights in his own soul evolved and grew hand in hand with his understanding of current Israeli society. His growing religious observance and spirituality provided him with a most complete view of Man's inner and outer worlds and the flow between these two. Moreover, it seemed to him that his own personal development and growing understandings were quite likely part of a pattern, a link in the millennia-long chain of Jewish development. Accordingly, his own emergence (and that of many others) from behind the Shadow of the Holocaust through religious observance and spirituality perhaps somewhat preceded similar developments in Jewish and Israeli society.

As a physician, I have always felt much honored, privileged and humbled to hear patients' medical histories and personal stories, and Moses P's story is just one of such. From an early stage in my medical career I was aware that I gained and grew from the interaction with my patients at least as much as they received from me. Gradually, I was able to articulate these thoughts. Although I at first felt some shame, as if I was cheating my patients, as if I had to be a perfect physician and solely outwardly oriented to heal my patients. I remembered the uncertainty principle from quantum mechanics, which states that the plain observation and measurement of objects changes those. Therefore, there was a scientific basis for my feeling that interaction with my patients affected them, but me too. Subsequently, with more personal growth, I came to understand that an emotionally uninvolved, mechanical physician would be an inefficient one. Moreover, physicians, like every other person choose their occupation because they have to undergo some personal development related to that profession. If a physician, or any person in any occupation believes he is entirely altruistic, purely oriented to give to persons and causes, he is either lacking insight or just simpleminded. Life is like commerce: we give in order to obtain. The plain gain is money, but the greater gain is social, emotional and spiritual.

I gained two important insights from the long relationship with Moses P. First, as Dr. Abulafia observed in his wonderful book "On the verge of Eden" the dialectic approach is less fruitful than the dialogue one. When Moses with much embarrassment expressed his feelings of professional and personal inadequacy and worthlessness - these feelings were ostentatiously at the bottom of his hyperactivity, providing him with a sense of being relevant and needed - I was astounded and tried to counter his feelings with arguments and proof. "Moses", I told him, "you are the epitome of a successful professional, much respected and sought after by your patients, at the top of your career, with a good salary, your students and residents greatly appreciate your teaching and you are a declared role model". He wanly smiled and for a brief moment appreciated my argument, but quickly fell back into despondency. There was evidently something inside that needed healing. So over time, as both of us grew, we tried the dialogue approach. "Of course", I told him, "you feel worthless. All men are in essence nothing but 70% water and very little substance. We live but briefly and fear the suffering that awaits many people before their death. We as physicians know: maybe one reason we chose our occupation was to get a better handle on our fear of death. You are to be *commended* that you feel worthless. In fact, so many people exude self-confidence, while inside their feelings may be quite opposite, or should be so. The Torah teaches that self confidence ("with my talents and abilities I have done all these great things") is just a misplaced sign of pride. Rather, we are taught, we should acknowledge and be thankful that God (or nature, if you are a non-believer) bestowed you with those characteristics which enabled you to become and do what you do. Our greatest Prophet Moses, your namesake, is described in the Torah as the most modest of all men on earth. One may and should ask how come? He was the great leader who performed miracles, led the Jewish people out of Egypt and spoke directly to God as no person before or after has done. His modestly derived from the fact that he did not deny his abilities, but knew they were *given* to him. His capabilities were not of his own making, like the Pharaoh in Exodus believed, who considered himself God who had created the Nile and everything else. Moreover, Moses knew that these capabilities were given to him not for his own pleasure, but in order *to do his task and duty*. At the first and crucial encounter between Moses and God at the burning bush, which did not turn to ashes, Moses actively resisted the task given to him, putting forth various arguments why he was not the right man for this job. Only begrudgingly and after quite some coercion, did Moses accept the task given to him. Maybe feelings of inadequacy led him believe to be incapable for the task ahead and someone else would be better qualified; possibly he preferred a pastoral life as shepherd. However, even from this little episode, you, Moses P and I too may obtain relevant insights. Man evidently does not know his task on earth. He is guided by a mix of desire and environmental forces. Moses knew what God planned for him, because He told him so and even then Moses resisted. We, lesser beings, have to guess our task by observing what Life had brought to us – and like Moses, resist and believe that we are destined for something else, a process accompanied by much dissatisfaction and unhappiness. In the Torah we observe how Moses, a shepherd of sheep and goats, who evidently stuttered and felt unworthy, ultimately accepted the task given to him, grew into it and turned into the most accomplished prophet of all times. Personal happiness is not and should not be the object of our endeavors: rather, we should do our tasks and satisfaction may be the natural byproduct."

The second major insight I gained from this long-standing relationship with Moses P is that a stint of psychotherapy maybe very useful for almost *every* individual. Every person carries a bag with unsolved emotional issues, which subconsciously steer his thought, talk and behavior. Our colleagues at work, our friends and especially our spouses know our idiosyncrasies, while these often remain hidden from us within our shadow (C.G. Jung's terminology). We grow by introspection and for a successful process most people need a partner, a spouse and occasionally a professional guide. Psychotherapy should help take care of old, unsolved and partially solved issues. However, beyond psychology is spiritual growth. I do not doubt the possibility of non-religious spiritual growth (see e.g. Chapter 2. Making sense of suffering: The baby with end stage renal disease, and others stories); but religious spirituality provides vastly wider and higher opportunity for growth. Moses P started his personal voyage as non-observant, hovering between atheism and a feeling that there "might be something else". He gained spiritual insights, such as that the generation of his parents preferred to be silent about the Holocaust, almost as if embarrassed that they had survived, while the real heroes were those who had not. Moreover, most survivors did not have hero stories to tell, but mostly ones of a struggle for personal survival, many of which seemed banal. Life can seem banal, even evil can seem banal, as Arendt indicated in the title of her book on Eichmann. Books and movies can provide a source for personal spiritual growth and Moses P had used these extensively during his younger years. However, he really "took off" after gradually becoming more religiously observant and through persistent study of ancient Jewish sources, bible and Talmud and multiple commentaries. Study of the biblical stories he knew superficially, provided ever deeper insight into Man's soul, including his own.

Chapter 12: Chronic fatigue syndrome: A case for complimentary medicine

Over the years, many patients have come to my infectious disease clinic because of chronic fatigue in order to obtain a second, third of fourth opinion. Most are in their twenties or thirties, although a few have been older. According to the medical literature, this condition may affect up to 5% of the population. Physical symptoms may vary, but the core complaint appears to be excessive tiredness during the daytime and inability to function appropriately. Many, although not all sleep many hours during the night, occasionally with naps during the day, but nonetheless feel without energy to go about their usual activities. The American Medical Association has issued a case definition in order to assist physicians to make the diagnosis, but in spite of extensive research no specific biological markers have been identified. Family physicians refer their patients to a rheumatologist if there is a component of bone and joint pains, in which instance the diagnosis usually becomes fibromyalgia; or alternatively, to an infectious disease consultant if there was a febrile episode at some point in the course of their fatigue. Epstein-Barr virus or Cytomegalovirus infection may produce an infectious mononucleosis like illness, not unlike influenza and while the vast majority recovers within a few days, a tail of listlessness and fatigue occurs in some, which may last several weeks or rarely months. Most of these patients bring along a pack of laboratory results, reports of imaging tests, ultrasound, CT scan and even MRI.

My approach to these patients has invariably been from the bottom up, starting with a detailed medical history, thorough physical examination and review of all laboratory tests. Although fatigue appears to be the most significant complaint in most patients, many have additional symptoms, leading to a differential diagnosis which differs from one patient to the other. Most patients have been seen repeatedly by their family physicians as well as by multiple consultants and both sides become increasingly frustrated. I always address their frustration, but first try to rule out a bio-medical source of their symptoms, such as malignancy or a collagen disease. In my report to their referring physician, I often suggest complementary tests to rule out those possible medical conditions. Although quite early in the consultation my intuition announces that there is no biomedical issue, I proceed according to the rules I was taught in medical school and which I continue to teach to my residents and students.

However, I never leave it at that and try to obtain a psycho-social history as detailed as the patient is willing to provide. Each person has a bag of memories, including unpleasant ones, some of which are raw and only partially digested. In many people, some past events were so traumatic, that even though there is no apparent causative connection with their presenting syndrome, they could benefit from appropriate professional assistance. Others actually ascribe the onset of their current illness to certain events in their personal, family or professional life. I usually conclude by suggesting to the patient that his syndrome is evidently not amenable to a simple solution, such as a doctor's prescription of a medication, which the patient would swallow. In fact, modern medicine has a range of medications, which one could easily prescribe, such as non steroidal anti-inflammatory agents, steroids, antidepressants and anxiolytics, but I believe patients are badly served with these drugs. Some of their symptoms would perhaps be alleviated, definitely not all and side effects would accrue and complicate matters. I never imply or suggest that my patient's problems are a figment of his imagination or are "from their head." Rather, the doctor, having concluded that there is no major biomedical illness needs to step aside in all humility because he cannot tell what is wrong and how to reduce his patient's suffering. He may provide hope by suggesting a new, possibly exciting direction. He can encourage his patient to take control of his own life, start on a voyage of discovery, a trip in uncharted territory. Although frightening and most would prefer to get along with their usual life, there is evidently no alternative. Moreover, this journey may turn out to be the most rewarding of their life, in which they may and are likely to discover parts of their real self and destiny.

According to their unique personal characteristics I have referred these patients for professional guidance to a great variety of directions, such as acupuncture, homoeopathy, reflexology, chiropractics, holistic pulsing, religious counseling, a dancing course, and others, almost invariably in combination with psychotherapy. It pays to inquire regarding practitioners of complementary and alternative medicine; although physicians cannot assess the professional ability of these practitioners, it is not too difficult to learn about the courses they have taken, their experience, the professional environment they have created, the standing among their patients, as well as satisfaction expressed by their patients regarding the care they received.

According to the medical literature, for each doctor's visit there are one and a half visits to a practitioner in complementary medicine. Modern medicine does not view these modes of therapy too kindly. The more liberal and open minded ascribe the success of complementary medicine to a placebo effect, which holds that up to 30% of any medication or mode of therapy has some positive effect even if entirely devoid of an active ingredient. However, the majority dismiss complementary medicine as quack or even fraudulent, its practitioners charging a sizeable fee per hour, which is often larger than their own per hour salary. They may express bitterness and anger, because they themselves have had to study many years and pass difficult examinations in order to obtain their license to practice, while many of the practitioners of complementary medicine have taken a course of whatever dubious nature and may start their business. Indeed, the field includes a range of very respectable people, some of who are physicians themselves and others, who have spent years studying and acquiring therapeutic skills, which are not taught in regular medical schools. Of course, there are practitioners, whose training experience has been very limited and who could do more harm than good. However, the bottom line is that general society does not agree with how modern medicine looks at complementary medicine. People of all sectors of society use complementary medicine, often in concert with regular medicine and usually without telling their doctor because the latter might dismiss that and possible them as well. Not only poorly educated, gullible people use complementary medicine. It is especially the richer and often better educated who do so, as these services are all private and mostly not covered by insurance plans. This is an awkward situation in which the professional sector of physicians dismisses the majority of society who uses complementary medicine. Majorities are not always right, but quite possibly the professionals could also miss something of real relevance. Doctors quote scientific studies of complementary medicine, which generally do not show objective evidence of effectiveness.

Sara P, the wife of Dr. Moses P described in the previous chapter was a real scientist, unlike her physician husband. Medicine is after all a profession, acquired at a trade/medical school; although based on exact sciences, the practice of medicine also extensively relies on psycho-social sciences. Sara had attended outstanding university programs and obtained a PhD degree in physics and pursued a successful career in research. However, following the birth of her children she experienced extended periods of post partum depressive moods, the first indication of a gathering cloud. Over the course of two decades she developed increasing emotional distress, sleep disorder and irritability, as well as bone and joint aches and digestive problems. Her husband being a family physician, they saw prominent specialists in various fields, ranging from rheumatology and immunology to endocrinology, who performed many tests but could not diagnose any biomedical problem. After much initial resistance she went to see a psychiatrist who prescribed an antidepressant and suggested that she would be alright within a few weeks. However, weeks, months and years passed, with psychotherapy and multiple psychiatric medications, while depression and desperation increased. Her ability to function at home, socially and professionally decreased and she had to discontinue her career as research scientist. Although suicidal ideation plagued her incessantly, day and night, she mustered with supreme determination the will to keep her family together and refrain from suicide. She wished to fight it through, whatever it takes, for "here stops the bug", with which she indicated her belief that suicide would only create further psychological distress for her children.

Sara, like her husband, was the descendent of holocaust survivors. Although her father, his parents and siblings all were hidden by righteous gentiles, her mother was the only survivor of her family. Sara's youth was marked by her mother's depressions and inability to function, common symptoms of Holocaust survivors with which the medical and psychiatric community at the time were unable to cope appropriately. In addition, each family has its own psycho-social peculiarities and Sara's parents had theirs too, on top of the Holocaust related issues. Indeed, Sara and her husband eventually realized that most and probably all Jews are descendants from generations of various Holocausts' survivors. The list only starts with that most outrageous of all, the wholesale genocide methodically organized by one of the "most advanced cultures" of all time. However, it goes back through endless pogroms; the Chmielnicki/Kozak sacking of countless eastern European Jewish communities and murder of some hundred thousand Jews in the 17th century; the Expulsion and forced conversion of remaining Spanish Jewry at the conclusion of the 15th century; the systematic torture and murder of countless Jews conducted by the Inquisition over many centuries; the wholesale murder of countless Jews and destruction of Jewish communities by the Crusaders; back to the oppression and misconduct of the Romans during centuries of rule of the Holy Land, including the destruction of the Second Temple and expulsion of the Jews from their land. Survivors must all have been emotionally scarred by the traumas of their times, families and communities, and many were survivors of multiple disasters. Their children and grandchildren all carry the impacts of these scars, which depth we can only surmise by looking at current second generation survivors of the Nazi Holocaust. Sara's determination "to fight it through" is all the more remarkable because of the intractability and depth of her depression and her psychiatrist's assessment that her personal background suggested that she would never attain complete cure and would require lifetime therapy.

Painstakingly, Sara set out to reclaim her life, entered uncharted territory, with no one to show the way or even promise a remote chance of a successful outcome. She only had her own intuition to guide her. Modern medicine had utterly failed her and left her on the brink of the abyss. However, Divine providence guided her, which she only later recognized as such. Gradually, she put together her own team of therapists, the first of whom was a reflexologist, who made her realize the connection between physical ailment and emotional distress. In addition, he helped her grow beyond emotional and psychological limits. When Sara started having various spiritual experiences she knew she was onto something entirely new, which gave her a first glimmer of hope. Eventually this led to understanding of the crucial importance of careful observance of the Torah's precepts (mitzvoth) for the spiritual stability and growth of every Jew. A dedicated Hassidic Rabbi, the second person on her team of therapists, guided her during those first steps and helped her appreciate ancient Jewish sources of incredible wisdom and insights into the soul of man.

The third person on her team was an outstanding therapist of classical homoeopathy, a branch that is truly alternative to modern medicine. This elderly woman, a medical doctor by training, gave her faith in herself as well in that homoeopathy could help her and with time to achieve complete cure. Over time Sara received various homoeopathic remedies, to be vigorously shaken before consumption. Modern medicine ridicules these remedies, because they are diluted to many times below the number of Avogadro, the dilution below which no molecules can be solvated in water. Modern medications are prescribed in small amounts, milligrams or at most grams and they positively affect our body's systems. Homoeopathic reasoning holds that the higher the titration, up to many times below Avogadro's number, the more potent the remedy. These effects have been observed in multiple anecdotal cases, in which patients with similar ailments received different remedies, individually matched for each person. Entire textbooks have been written in the last two centuries, since Hahnemann pioneered this approach. His observation that a disease could be cured with a highly diluted remedy producing a similar disease pattern was radically different from modern medicine, which prescribes medications that oppose the disease phenomena. For example, high fever is often treated with paracetamol, which induces perspiration and a drop in temperature. Homoeopathic medical schools abounded in Europe and the US up till the beginning of the 20th century and all closed with the rising successes of modern medical sciences. However, homoeopathy has continued to flourish in the Indian subcontinent and has subsequently made a comeback in various western societies.

Over time, Sara gradually improved. Her depression subsided, suicidal ideation disappeared and physical symptoms gradually abated. After several years, she discontinued follow-up one after the other with her therapeutic team. She continued to be active in her personal and family life and even resumed highly productive research activities, several years after she had given up all scientific endeavors and had been sure that this would be definite. During these years, her husband gradually gained confidence in his wife's miraculous cure. However, as a physician, he felt astounded and shaken. After all, modern medicine had been unable to cure or even alleviate his wife's suffering, while a combination of alternative and complementary therapists had affected a complete cure. During our frequent conversations, Moses P shared with me his own concerns and suffering on account of his wife protracted ailments; and how she gradually but completed recovered with homoeopathy, reflexology, guided imagery, maintaining a natural diet and through becoming religiously observant. Each of these therapies probably contributed something to the overall outcome, but homoeopathy was the persistent thread throughout the entire process. Was it the therapeutic effect of the interaction with the therapist? Possibly this component contributed, but Sara had been treated by very kind, wise and professional psychotherapists, reducing the possibility that the cure had been effected by this factor only. This reasoning led to the near inconceivable conclusion that the homoeopathic remedy included some really therapeutic action, in spite of the fact that it could not include an active molecule save water. When a course opened for homoeopathy for physicians, Moses P enrolled and he convinced me to join him. During four-hour weekly sessions over three years we studied the theory of homoeopathy as expounded by Hahnemann in his Organon, an interesting piece of medical philosophy, which confronted us with the fact that there is no philosophy of modern medicine, safe a pragmatic, empiric approach. This was made accessible by a teacher, who was a graduate medical doctor by himself, before studying homoeopathy. The other major component of the course consisted of the study of homoeopathic remedies. This proved to be enormously challenging to our medical minds, primed by physiology, pathology and other basic sciences. Homoeopathic remedies have a profile active on various levels, physical and mental, and no anatomic or physiologic common pathway can be found. The remedies were taught by a superb teacher and homoeopath, who was not a medical doctor and she was able to convey the essence of it. Remedies and diseases have a symbolic underlying pattern. E.g., if a person has a cramped, constricted view of life, brought on in part by childhood circumstances, not only his outlook on life is narrow, but he may suffer from irritable bowel syndrome, as well as obstructed arteries causing heart disease and ischemic legs. These insights were radically different from what we had learned in medical school. Although infections were brought on by infecting microorganisms, we never knew why upon exposure to a particular organism one person would fall ill, while the next did not. "Host factors" were evidently involved, things we could not identify or quantify. Homoeopathy suggested a causative role for emotional, psychological factors.

One fascinating event occurred during one of these sessions. The topic of the session was Kent's Repertory of the Homoeopathic Materia Medica, a lengthy discourse of the remedies. Leafing through the introduction, Moses P came upon an anecdote, describing how Kent, a graduate of a regular medical school and practitioner in the US at the onset of the 20th century, became interested in homoeopathy. His wife had fallen ill with a protracted and debilitating illness and his physician colleagues had been unable to prescribe a cure or alleviate her suffering. In desperation, they turned to homoeopathy and his wife evidently made a complete recovery.

We have not become practicing homoeopaths. However, Moses P is happy with his wife's recovery, while I myself feel much more comfortable referring patients to alternative and complementary medicine if their ailments cannot be diagnosed or do not seem amenable to therapy within the biomedical realm. Stated differently, there may be four broad levels of medicine. The lowest level is occupied by naturopathy, which attempts to cure ailments, or prevent disease a priori by paying attention to food. Servan-Schreiber, a US-based neuro-psychiatrist of French extraction presented a lot of research as well opinions on food in his best-selling book "Anti-Cancer". His results and opinions appear to converge with those of naturopathy. The second level, one step up, is occupied by modern medicine, which, after disease has manifested in physical signs, concerns itself with diagnosis and treatment in biological terms. One step up is homoeopathy and possible some other forms of alternative and complementary medicine as well. This level is on the one hand more remote from the physical manifestations of disease, while on the other hand closer to the possible emotional, psychological, and perhaps spiritual sources of illness. The fourth and highest level is occupied by the Torah, the study of which, together with a life conducted according to its precepts (mitzvoth) should ideally prevent all disease according to Exodus 15:26: "He (God) said: If you vigilantly obey the voice of the Almighty, your God, and do what is upright in His eyes, give ear to His commandments, and preserve all His statutes, [then] every sickness that I brought upon Egypt I will not bring upon you, for I am God who heals you". The very concept that physical and even mental disease could possibly derive from emotional and spiritual dis-ease is entirely foreign to modern medicine and most of its practitioners would scoff at the idea. However, to me it has become abundantly clear after thirty years in practice that true and complete healing of physical illness involves – in combination with modern medicine – a complementary component, where the patient rises above his physical ailment to come into closer contact with his spiritual being.

Chapter 13: Chronic urinary tract infection? What if ovaries could speak?

Jocelyn Greece was a 70 year woman, who came for an infectious disease consultation accompanied by Henry, her 73 year old husband. They were recent immigrants from France, where they were born and had lived their entire lives. They had three children, all married and the last one had moved to Israel some ten years earlier. It felt only natural for the elderly couple to follow their children and especially their grandchildren, after both had retired from their respective careers, she as a high school teacher and he as a successful businessman. Their English was fluent, tinged with a distinguished sounding French accent. Both looked relaxed and comfortable together.

Jocelyn had always been in excellent health. Up to the present she did not take regular medications for any chronic ailment, like diabetes, hypertension, heart disease or hyperlipidemia. Jocelyn came to see me because of a new problem, which had been bothering her over the last year: recurrent, perhaps chronic urinary tract infection. While she explained her problem, her husband retrieved a neatly organized file, which included results of at least fourteen urine cultures, out of which common urinary pathogens had been isolated, mostly E. coli and occasionally Proteus. She had received multiple courses of antimicrobial drugs over the last year, some of which had given her significant side effects, such as nausea, rash and a vaginal yeast infection. Worse, the infection did not appear to clear and a few days after discontinuation of an antibiotic course her symptoms would recur. The pathogens had become increasingly resistant to antibiotics, and the last course consisted of the very broad spectrum drug ertapenem, which she received during a five day admission to another hospital. I wondered whether she was acutely ill when she was admitted, which she denied: the antibiotic which she needed to cover the organism isolated from her urine had to be given intravenously and was very expensive. Accordingly, the hospital demanded admission to recoup for the incurred expense of the drug.

Could Jocelyn please describe her symptoms? She readily obliged, described her complaints in crisp, well defined sentences. She felt lower abdominal pains, which would come and go, usually pretty sharp, occasionally dull in character. The pain might occur every few days, up to several times per day and might stay between several minutes to several hours. She denied nausea or diarrhea: she had regular bowel movements, without any recent change. When the pain appeared, she usually went to pass urine, but urination was not accompanied by any particular unpleasant sensation, nor did it provide relief from the abdominal pain. She did not have to pass urine more often than usual and she denied stress incontinence, an unpleasant but common symptom in elderly women. In addition to the urine cultures, she had done an abdominal ultrasound and CT scan, both of which had been entirely normal.

Urinary tract infections are among the most common infections family physicians, internists and infectious disease consultants encounter. Although they occur at all ages and both sexes, more than 99% of all cases occur in women of reproductive age. Onset of sexual relations is an oft recognized precipitating factor, and this association has lead to the term honeymoon cystitis. In spite of the fact that almost all women engage in sexual activity, only a small fraction suffers from urinary tract infections for unknown reason. The usual triad of symptoms consists of dysuria, a burning sensation during urination; frequency, the need to pass urine much more often than usual; and urgency, the need to rush to the bathroom or else lose control – only to pass a few drops. In the majority of cases of cystitis, the most common manifestation of urinary tract infection, there is no or only a little elevated temperature. In only a small percentage of cases the infection may ascend to involve the kidneys, a condition called pyelonephritis, causing flank pain, high fever and chills, and hospitalization for intravenous therapy is urgently needed. The laboratory diagnosis of urinary tract infection consist of obtaining a urine sample, firstly for culture in order to isolate the causative organisms and determine its susceptibility to various antimicrobials; and, secondly for urinalysis, to determine the presence of white cells, an indicator of infection, and nitrites, breakdown products of bacteria.

After Jocelyn and her husband had related their complaints, I carefully reviewed the laboratory results they had brought along. Although out of the majority of cultures a common urinary pathogen had been isolated, I was immediately struck by the fact that only in one of these samples the urinalysis revealed nitrites. So I started my discussion with my patient and her husband by saying that I would first review with them these urine results and their significance, to be followed by discussing her symptoms and the (doubtful) relation between the cultures and her symptoms, then examine her and finally try to put everything together. So what was the relevance of these urine cultures, what did they mean? The fact that no nitrites were present strongly suggested sampling error, indicating that significant contamination of the specimen had occurred while it was being collected. This is especially common in women, because the urethra opens onto the mucous membrane covering the perineum and the opening is covered by the major labia. When women pass urine it touches the perineal mucous membrane and skin of the labia, all of which are colonized by bowel flora, organisms deriving from the large intestine. Urine specimens are cultured on media favoring bacterial growth; therefore, if the urine specimen contains any organism the culture will reveal growth. It is therefore of crucial importance that prior to obtaining a urine specimen the woman is instructed regarding appropriate sampling. This starts by using two fingers of one hand to spread the major labia and expose the opening of the urethra and keep it exposed until the collection of the specimen is completed. Subsequently, the exposed urethral opening needs to be cleaned with a provided antiseptic wipe, after which the woman should start passing urine. Only after the urine stream has become steady she should use her second hand to pass the provided sterile canister into the urine stream in order to collect several milliliters of urine and remove the canister before the urine streams weakens and stops, and only then she may relax her other hand's fingers from the labia. After carefully closing the cover of the sterile canister, without touching the rim or contents, may this specimen provide relevant information. "No one", said Jocelyn, "had ever explained anything like this to me". Moreover, she had never spread her labia away from the urine stream while obtaining specimens. Now she and her husband understood that the absence of nitrites indicated that the organisms, isolated from her urine specimens, indicated that these had resulted from a few skin colonizers rather than from multiple bacteria that had been sitting and growing in her urinary bladder, which would have been accompanied by bacterial breakdown and nitrite production.

We subsequently turned to the major issue: her complaints. I reminded her that I first had asked for a detailed account of her symptoms, before relating the common "triad of symptoms" that were the hallmark of urinary tract infection in the vast majority of patients, and women in particular. However, occasionally symptoms could be different, as what happens in babies, producing diarrhea; or in elderly, dement and bedridden patients, who unfortunately cannot express themselves verbally and signs of general deterioration, such as apathy and lack of appetite are common. However, Jocelyn was perfectly able to express herself. Her major symptom was misery on account of lower abdominal pains, occasionally of sudden, shooting character and occasionally they were dull and staying for hours. These pain had accompanied her most of the days over the last year. Although she associated these pains with urinary tract infection, urination was not accompanied by pain or burning, nor did it lead to relief of symptoms. Her appetite was normal, her weight stable and her bowel movements regular and unchanged, which, any of which if abnormal, could have indicated an intestinal source of her complaints. Interestingly, only the one intravenous course of antibiotics she received was associated with a temporary improvement of her lower abdominal pains. This improvement could have been due to the antibiotics, but, I suggested, could also be due to the enforced several days of rest in hospital...

Her physical examination was entirely normal, except that of the lower abdomen. Palpation revealed exquisite tenderness in both lower quadrants, localized in two small zones, each perhaps five by five centimeters, about ten centimeters from the midline. I asked Jocelyn and her husband whether she knew what structures could be behind those localized pains, and we made the "differential diagnosis" together. They got as far as mentioning the bowel, perhaps diverticulae; I added the ovaries. The patient and her husband exchanged a knowing look, the significance of which I could not even guess at the time. From the abdominal CT scan which the patient had undergone, we already knew that there was no major abdominal problem, including diverticulae of the colon, or a growth involving the ovaries. She mentioned that she had recently undergone a pelvic examination and that no gynecological source of her abdominal pains was found.

I tried to put everything together. Jocelyn suffered from lower abdominal pains, which had been bothering her for a year. She and her doctor had ascribed these pains to urinary tract infections, but repeat antibiotic courses had not solved the problem. Rather, she had developed multiple side effects, while the organisms growing out of the urine cultures were increasingly resistant to antibiotics. The urine cultures could all have been false positive on account of sampling error. Were urinary tract infections the source of her lower abdominal pains? I doubted so, because of the lack of urinary symptoms, absence of nitrites in the urine and lack of response to antibiotics. What else could it be? I had two advantages above Jocelyn's previous physicians: first, the symptoms had already been present for a year, within which she had not lost weight or developed additional symptoms, which could have indicated an underlying serious illness. Second, she had had blood tests and a CT scan, which were entirely normal and therefore reassuring.

I could not possibly dismiss Jocelyn and her husband with this. If it was not a urinary tract infection, then what was it? I mentioned to Jocelyn that medicine often is an exercise in modesty. Hospital based physicians are used to see patients with severe physical illnesses. Community based physicians, on the other hand, frequently encounter patients with multiple somatic complaints for which no underlying physical explanation can be found. Some of these patients keep returning to their physicians, undergo expensive and extensive evaluation, which still does not reveal any particular physical ailment, leading to significant frustration in both patient and physician. Should we actually or figuratively point a finger at our patient's head and suggest that their symptoms are a product of imagination or emotional instability? Such behavior would be both crude and counter-productive and I subscribe to a more skillful approach. I prefer to explain that successive practitioners of modern medicine have evidently been unable to make a diagnosis and/or provide effective treatment for their symptoms. However, fortunately no evidence was found of a serious physical illness. Rather than insist that modern medicine make a definite diagnosis and prescribe a curative medicine, I try to reassure my patients and simultaneously empower them. Instead of accepting the doctor's verdict that everything is all right, except the fact that the patients continue to suffer from their symptoms, they should be encouraged to actively engage their symptoms, analyze their symbolic significance and work through them. Practitioners of complementary medicine are much better suited to work with these issues than physicians, including psychiatrists.

With Jocelyn I discussed several variations of body-mind medicine. I knew from experience that young people and especially women are more open minded regarding complementary medicine, while elderly and especially male patients are especially reluctant to try anything that involves work with emotions and introspection. Baby boomers are somewhere in between. With Jocelyn, my intuition told me to carefully avoid the option of psychotherapy. Rather, I briefly mentioned three different methods that had a common theme: they use guided imagery to encounter and possibly cure a symptomatic body part. First, considering Jocelyn's French background, I referred her to Lise Bourbeau, a Canadian French speaking therapist, who has written several books about her ideas and treatment technique, including "Listen to your body, your best friend on earth." In this and other books Bourbeau discusses her insights regarding the possible symbolic meaning of various organs and their ailments. Second, I referred her to Brandon Bays, an American therapist who wrote several books, including The Journey, in which she described her own inner journey to conquer a huge tumor of her uterus without surgery or chemotherapy. Bays teaches her healing technique at seminars and has trained many therapists, including licensed psychotherapists who use her technique as part of their repertoire. Finally, I discussed with her Holistic Pulsing, a technique developed by Tovi Browning, a graduate of a British school of naturopathy. The therapist gently rocks the patient, lying on a couch and helps the patient make appropriate connections between various mind issues and body parts or zones. The three techniques and probably many similar ones, help the patient relax by breathing exercises, and then guide the closed-eyed patient through free-floating associations or imagery to encounter their symptoms, try to reach their emotional basis and heal them. Perhaps Jocelyn would like to become more active at discovering the source of her lower abdominal pain and solve her problem without resorting to modern medicine, which anyway appeared to be unable to cure it?

I wondered aloud whether all this sounded like new-ageism to Jocelyn. If so, I mentioned that the Bible was full of references to emotional and especially spiritual problems as source of physical illness. The one illness described in exhaustive detail in the Pentateuch is leprosy, which the sages unanimously see as punishment for slander. I recounted the story of king Uziah, who had the audacity to enter the Holy Temple and burn a frankincense offering (described in detail in chapter 10: Leprosy: a case of drug toxicity only). Perhaps the most specific Biblical sentence on physical illness as an expression of an underlying spiritual problem is in Exodus (15: 26): "If you vigilantly obey the voice of the Lord your God and do what is upright in His eyes, give ear to His commandments, and preserve all His statutes, then every sickness that I brought upon Egypt I will not bring upon you, for I am God who heals you".

As usual, I supplied Jocelyn with a written summary for her referring physician. I recommended obtainment of a urine culture and urinalysis if symptoms recurred, and accentuated the importance of appropriate sampling. My patient and her husband were definitely reassured by the extensive and exhaustive consultation. Nonetheless, I felt uncomfortable, as if I had distanced myself too much from physical medicine. Perhaps my patient had not been able to follow the latter part of our discussion, regarding body-mind therapy, which is definitely not something that modern medicine advertizes. Perhaps the idea that some unsolved or partially solved emotional issue could be at the root of her abdominal pains felt threatening to her. Fortunately, several days later the family physician called in order to discuss his patient in further detail. He felt "at a dead end" when he referred her to me. We discussed the lack of diagnostic certainty regarding urinary tract infections as explanation for her abdominal pains. Rather than leave the patient and her doctor in limbo, I briefly mentioned the issue of empowering patients to move from being passive (waiting for their doctor to solve their problems) to become actively involved in the process of understanding and curing their symptoms. Physicians are rightly reluctant to do so; firstly, because we are loath to miss a diagnosis and rather follow our patients, do more tests and obtain expert opinions. Secondly, most physicians have not received formal training about complementary and alternative medicine, either have strong opinions about it (usually dismissing it out of hand as unproven baloney) or have not given it much thought, in spite of the fact that many of their patients make use of it simultaneously with modern medicine. However, once we have applied our best medical knowledge and have not been able to reach a reasonable diagnosis and/or solved our patient's symptoms, we should be able to confess our medical limits and be confident enough to help the patient consider complimentary medicine. The family physician greatly appreciated our talk. I felt better myself, but was still not entirely reassured.

Several months later Jocelyn called; she wished to see me and ask me a specific question. Although I did not expect so from her phone call, she brought Henry along. Jocelyn started out by saying that our one-time meeting had set into motion a long dormant process. Some twenty five years earlier, she and her husband had gone though a midlife marital crisis. A downturn in the French economy had adversely affected Henry's business and he was near bankruptcy. He had built his agricultural export business from scratch and he had always felt pride to be a good provider for his family. However, his business had become his temple, where he met colleagues and where important financial transactions took place. He derived a sense of meaning and raison d'être that according to his wife's feeling went way beyond that of most men. He had become a workaholic, usually spending twelve to fourteen hours each day in his business. Accordingly, Jocelyn, who worked as a school teacher, raised their three children almost singlehandedly. They had lived a secular lifestyle and many of her female friends were French middle-class intellectuals. Together they commiserated about their empty marriages and the estrangement between husbands and wives on account of the husbands forever foraging in the wider world and not spending quality time with their wives and children. The near crash of his firm brought Henry to his knees. He developed incapacitating migraines and became depressed to the point that he was unable to get to work several times each week. His irritability became a severe problem to his wife and teenage children. Like all marriages they had had their ups and downs. Nonetheless, in spite of Henry being a workaholic he had always been a faithful husband and respectful to his wife and she had, therefore, never seriously considered a divorce. At this crisis period in their life, Jocelyn started missing one or two menstrual periods. As she was 46 years old at the time, she was not unduly surprised and ascribed the irregularity to early onset menopause or perhaps the current stressful period. However, when morning sickness development she went to see her gynecologist who quickly confirmed that she was pregnant. Jocelyn was flabbergasted. They had always been careful about birth control. Moreover, sexual relations had diminished considerably over the last few years, reflecting the estrangement between the couple. However, there were fond of each other, respected each other and had not entirely separated.

While at her gynecologist's office she called Henry at home and demanded that he take a taxi and immediately join her because of a medical emergency. Henry had been in bed with migraine, miserable, nauseous and vomiting. His wife's fearful, panicky voice over the phone galvanized him. From being miserable and withdrawn within himself, his mindfulness turned completely outward, towards his wife who evidently needed him urgently. His migraine subsided, color returned to his face and he again became the energetic robust man Jocelyn had married long ago. He shortly joined her, was informed of the situation, his wife being ten weeks pregnant. Their options consisted of interrupting the pregnancy within the next ten days, or continuing the pregnancy with or without amniocentesis at twenty weeks of pregnancy to rule out chromosomal abnormality on account of Jocelyn's age. The next several days were like a dream, which transformed their lives. They discussed the pro's and con's of their options, the implications of each. Moreover, Henry expressed a considerateness for his wife's feelings and respect for her swinging emotional states that astounded and deeply touched her. Henry for his part was astonished by a deep sense of love for his wife that had been unavailable to him in years. They reached the same conclusion: this pregnancy had become a gift to transform their crisis time. It was therefore self evident that they would continue with it. Their teenage children were informed of the pregnancy and all were relieved to see their parents getting back to normalcy. Henry returned to his work with renewed vigor, after promising and sticking to his promise to make work days of not longer than nine hours and spend the weekends at home. They had yet to decide whether to have an amniocentesis at week twenty of pregnancy: Henry once actually mentioned to the gynecologist that he was not sure he would be able to tolerate the involved pain. Both he and Jocelyn were not sure they would be able to discontinue the pregnancy if the baby turned out to have Down syndrome. Their marriage had received an enormous boost as a result of this pregnancy: how could they consider terminating it?

They were spared the anguish of making this hard decision, but not another agony. When Jocelyn was sixteen weeks pregnant she suddenly developed lower abdominal pain and severe vaginal bleeding. On admission to hospital a fetal ultrasound revealed absence of heartbeat and she was diagnosed with spontaneous abortion. Because of continued bleeding she was rushed to the operating room. While one gynecologist tried to stop the source of bleeding a colleague stepped out to Henry. His wife's uterus had ruptured, probably at the site of the scar of a previous cesarean section and the uterus had to be removed to save her life. The doctor would like to know Henry's attitude regarding removal of the adnexa, the ovaries and salpinges, the tiny tubes leading from the ovaries to the uterus. Henry had never been particularly knowledgeable about the inner organs of women, but this was quickly remedied. What were the implications of leaving the adnexa alone, versus removing them? Removing the ovaries would prevent ovarian cancer. Leaving them would allow the continuation of hormonal production, although menstruation would not occur anyway due to absence of the uterus. Possibly, his wife would feel better and more feminine with the presence of functioning ovaries until they would atrophy within a few years. Henry was at a loss, the doctor refused to make a recommendation, so Henry eventually decided to leave the ovaries in place, with his wife's well being and well-feeling as the major argument. Joy recovered after an eventful hospitalization that lasted several weeks. The left ovaries and associated decision making process were mentioned once, but not further discussed.

Henry's business recovered. He stuck to his promises regarding a reasonable work week. Their family life improved significantly, as Henry and the children rallied around Jocelyn, who went back to teaching several months after the abortion. They organized a thanksgiving party at the local synagogue. They were profoundly thankful for the new lease on life they felt that the entire family had received. As often happens after crisis situations, they cherished life and each other more profoundly than before. Their social life increased, they started to attend concerts and for Jocelyn the most important of it all was the increased quality time they spent each week together, just talking about their lives and associated feelings. They felt changed for the better, matured beyond recognition. Although not religious, they spent more social time with other families attending the same synagogue. The local rabbi often stressed personal, social and Zionist issues in his talks with which they readily identified. The years passed, their children married and started building their own families and one after the other decided to move to Israel, positively influenced by their rabbi and negatively motivated by rising anti-Semitism in France. After Jocelyn and Henry joined their children, Jocelyn started to kindergarten two of her toddler grandchildren, five days each week.

Jocelyn stopped her animated monologue. Henry had been quiet all along, evidently spell bound while his wife related their story. Twice he made motions as if wanting to interrupt, once when his wife described his work habits and associated estrangement at home prior to the pregnancy, the other time when Jocelyn raised the operation and his decision to leave her ovaries in place. His eyes sparkled when Jocelyn described their new found energy and Henry's personal rebirth after the pregnancy. He looked at her with tears in his eyes, but remained silent. After the silence continued for a minute or so, I broke it and thanked Jocelyn for coming and sharing their story with me. "And now", I said, "You may want to raise the specific question which you mentioned over the phone". She indeed had a specific issue, but before raising it, she wanted to express her deep gratitude for the opportunity to just relate their personal story. It gave her an enormous sense of relief and satisfaction. The specific question had obviously to do with her ovaries. Her female productive organs had once saved their family from auto destruction and had elevated the parents and children to a higher, more spiritual level of living. It appeared that currently her ovaries, thankfully left behind by her husband's intuitive, but wise decision, were speaking up and demanding attention. She and Henry had discussed the possibility that her duties with her grandchildren were more demanding than her physiology would allow. However, they wished to get beyond that and explore their pasts, their present and especially their future lives. They wished to reread the events of their lives and derive meaning from each episode, until the very core of their personal and combined being. Could I please repeat the various options of complementary medicine I had mentioned at the final part of their first visit with me, as they had only been able to absorb part of that information. They intended to pursue their own path to self growth and heeling with a combination of two modalities, one for Jocelyn alone, the other for both of them together.

Chapter 14: Peyronie's disease: transforming weakness to strength.

The outpatient clinics in my specialty are scheduled for the afternoons, which allows one to first take care of hospitalized patients and urgent problems – and the afternoon hours are usually easier for out-patients as well. In the morning before clinics I usually review the names of patients for that afternoon's session. If necessary, I review the relevant files beforehand in order to be prepared, technically and psychologically. The schedule usually consists of a mix of new and follow-up patients. One particular day, several years ago, I saw a new name on the list, a Mr. Shneor Weisman[1], a name vaguely familiar to me, but even before getting to meet him I received an outside phone call announcing his arrival. I knew the caller: he was the well-known head of an office that refers patients to the "most appropriate doctor" for their medical problems. My caller wished to give me some background information regarding the new patient I would see that afternoon. Mr. Weisman was a wealthy Hassid, head of a chain of laundrinettes and philanthropist, who had made significant contributions to worthy goals. Mr. Weisman had consulted with the caller: he wished to see a physician, who could take care of "intimate and complicated" problems and, if needed, coordinate various disciplines. However, the patient had not disclosed his problems, so my caller was not certain these problems were within my field of expertise. If not, we would be in contact after the clinic visit in order to ascertain an appropriate referral.

When the patient entered my office I was immediately impressed with his modest, but dignified appearance. He was of median height, with a long beard and sideburns and wore black clothes and the hat typical of the Hassidic faction he was member of. I introduced myself, we shook hands and sat down for the interview. The first few seconds of a patient-doctor encounter often determine the degree of trust and quality of the subsequent relationship. In this instance I felt immediate rapport, we were on good track. Mr. Weisman – "please call me Shneor", which I did not – was at the time 58 years old, married and father of eight children, all of whom were married except the last one and of course he had multiple grandchildren. Who counts? He had God bless always been in excellent health. He was overweight, but not overtly obese. He had never been hospitalized and did not recall the last time he had seen a doctor. He paused for a moment for introspection, evidently considering how to present his

---

[1] The reader is reminded that although this narrative as all others in this book are based on true stories all identifying components have been entirely changed to protect privacy.

current problem. "God has given me a test. In the study of the Torah we discuss at length the ten tests Abraham received and how he overcame each with honor. We know that the stories of the Fathers are a sign and teaching to their descendants. Nonetheless, it is much easier to discuss someone else's predicaments and learn from them than actually experience such yourself. Moreover, *we* know the outcome of Abraham's quandaries, although he did not". He again reflected, before continuing: "The first mitswah (command) we were given in the Torah is to be fruitful and multiply. However, even after we have fulfilled this mitswah and even after your wife is not being able to conceive any longer, our sages encourage us to continue marital relations as long as our health permits". He glanced at me, as if asking whether I understood his point. I think I did: was this a problem of impotence? I nodded sympathetically to indicate that I had carefully followed his reasoning, but waited, hoping he would proceed. "About two months ago I felt some pain on the sides after intercourse. Pain is a tall word: it was more like heaviness or a burning sensation. It lasted for a few hours and passed. Over the next few weeks it has happened only once or twice again. However, I have noticed a certain deformity starting at the base near my belly and some new bending. God bless there has not been any problem with actual functioning. I have asked my wife and she admitted that there has been a "lesser degree of knowing", although this did not pose any problem to her. However, we have agreed I should see a doctor".

People who regularly study Torah are steeped in the biblical use of ultra-clean language. There are no coarse words for organs of proliferation. The actual act of procreation is termed "knowing", ever since Adam knew his wife, or at most "the use of one's bed". Since ancient times our sages have known and taught us that the use of clean language polishes us and generates a clean inner world and, vice versa, use of rude language roughens one's soul. With proper language, behavior and preparation marital intimacy becomes an act of holiness. My patient had described his predicament in clear, but circumspect terms and even without asking any questions or examining him I already knew the diagnosis. Nonetheless, I proceeded according to routine. I expressed appreciation for his trust and careful explanation. Upon my questioning he denied presence of diabetes, high blood pressure or heart disease; he had smoked cigarettes until his mid twenties, but not ever since; and he did not take any medications or drugs and had a glass of wine with the meals on Sabbath and Festivals only. The physical examination was unremarkable except for some abdominal overweight. On his penis I felt some subcutaneous nodules, which were slightly tender to palpation. In its flaccid condition no abnormal curvature could be detected.

If one enters curvature or bending of the penis in medical literature computer programs, especially if one crosses these terms with male dyspareunia or painful intercourse, the program quickly raises Peyronie's disease (PD). This condition was named after the French physician Francois de la Peyronie in 1741. His original description was one of "fibrous cavernositis preventing men from having normal ejaculation of semen". The disease is currently thought to affect between three and ten percent of men, usually in their late fifties or early sixties. Its prevalence appears to be rising, though this may be due to the fact that more men are seeking treatment for erectile dysfunction. Despite extensive research, much remains unknown about the origin and optimal treatment of the disease. PD is a localized connective tissue disorder of the penis leading to fibrosis, scarring and compromised ability of the soft tissue entitled tunica albuginea within the penis to fill with blood during arousal. According to one theory the immediate cause of fibrosis is thought to be ischemia and inflammation from repeated penile trauma or microtrauma. The resulting microvascular tears in this region lead to collagen deposition in the form of plaques. The unique appearance of PD during the patients' late fifties, when their wives may be in their early-mid fifties suggests a possible causal relationship with the women's menopause and associated decreased vaginal lubrication, which could lead to increased friction and microtrauma. Patients typically present with any of three complaints: a palpable plaque, a painful erection, and/or penile curvature. Penile curvature can in fact be so severe that it interferes with the ability to engage in intercourse. The disease undergoes a transition between two phases: an acute inflammatory phase and a chronic phase. Painful erections, developing penile curvature and nodule formation mark the acute inflammatory phase. This phase is self-limiting, typically lasting between six and eighteen months. Because the disease is evolving during this phase, the patient's pain, the degree of curvature and the size of the plaque may also undergo change. The chronic phase is characterized by minimal or no pain with stable nodule size and some degree of penile deformity.

Patients with PD are usually taken care of by urologists and family physicians, although I have encountered some cases in the sexually transmitted disease clinic during my fellowship in the US and more recently in my infectious disease clinic. The internist needs to rule out presence of an underlying systemic disease such as diabetes and hypertension, which may cause erectile dysfunction. The infectious disease consultant wishes to rule out presence of sexually transmitted diseases, but there appears to be no connection whatsoever between these and PD.

One of the advantages of medicine is that even the most complicated issues can be explained in simple wording that is readily accessible to most people. I gave my patient a brief overview of PD, its possible source and likely natural history. I tried to reassure him by stating that the disease is so common that he probably knew quite some men with the same condition – but not unexpectedly this did not provide much comfort. According to some reviews, up to thirty percent develop impotence. Even if the statistics were more encouraging, Mr. Weisman would have been concerned that perhaps he would be one of those experiencing bending that did not allow appropriate functioning. So he wondered what could be done to improve his chances. I told him I would review some common therapeutic options, but he would have to consult with an urologist because urologists are supposed to be up to date on this issue and PD is not within the field of expertise of infectious disease doctors.

According to the most recent reviews, which I downloaded from the computer, the treatment of PD is not clear at all. The protracted and variable course has made clinical research quite difficult. Most urologists start with oral medications, and according to need proceed with intraplaque injections and finally corrective surgery to facilitate intercourse. Various oral medications, such as vitamin E, colchicin and pentoxifylline have been tried in small studies, but few with consistent success. Oral pentoxifylline may be the most successful both in laboratory and clinical studies; the drug has been in use for many years for various other conditions, side effects are uncommon and it is cheap. Although topical creams have been used their effectiveness is unproven and therefore not recommended. Intralesional injections with verapamil or interferon may prevent further plaque formation and worsening of bending. There may also be room for combination treatment, with an oral drug and local injections. As mentioned, surgery is usually done only in patients, whose curvatures do not facilitate proper functioning.

Mr. Weisman looked at me carefully. "Thank you for your thorough explanation" he said. "Now, if this concerned your relative or even yourself, what would you do?" Indeed, Mr. Weisman had asked the ultimate and relevant question, the one which we always have to ask ourselves regarding our patients, especially concerning those who themselves are unable to consider the best therapeutic option. I actually love the question: rather than provide only the best technical advice, it transports the physician to the position of trusted and experienced adviser, who is asked to provide guidance with prudence and wisdom. I silently considered. The clinical studies that had been conducted with the various therapeutic options had been small, producing non consistent and therefore non-convincing results. Surgery at this point was out of the question because Mr. Weisman did not complain of functionality problems. Another option consisted of waiting and seeing. Finally, especially if Mr. Weisman decided on the latter option, he could chose on some form of complementary medicine, although I refrained from mentioning this option for now. My recommendation was simple, straightforward and without any reservation. "You have to see an expert urologist and have his opinion. Afterwards we may consider again". Mr. Weisman agreed provided I would recommend the name of the appropriate urologist and talk with him and he insisted on seeing me afterwards to discuss his options. How could I refuse a request of such overt trust?

Exactly one week later, Mr. Weisman was again on my clinic list. He had seen the urologist to whom he had been referred. As requested, I had called the urologist before the patient came to see him and afterwards the urologist called me to provide follow-up. He confirmed my diagnosis of PD. It looked like a moderately severe case of PD, because there was evidently bending of more than thirty degrees although there was as yet no interference with intercourse. He recommended combination treatment with vitamin E and pentoxifylline, as well as copious use of lubricant, but he was aware of the significant limitations in the urological literature regarding this or any treatment of PD. Although this urologist was not particularly religious he suggested that one should "hope, or pray" for a good outcome. I had had one week respite and was therefore more or less prepared when Mr. Weisman asked whether he should take the prescribed medications and was there any other recourse?

There are many more conditions for which modern medicine does not possess a therapy that has reasonable evidence to produce a favorable outcome. In such cases I stick to the most innocuous medication or treatment possible, even if evidence for efficacy is not conclusive. I am perfectly agreeable - and so are most patients - to accept the placebo effect, which states that in up to thirty percent of patients symptoms of any condition may improve with a medication devoid of an active ingredient. In addition, I try to gauge my patient's interest in the possible symbolic meaning of their symptoms or disease. If there is such an interest, I subsequently suggest some options that might be appealing to them. I am not an expert regarding alternative and complementary medicine (CAM), although I have talked in depth with several practitioners and have observed some modes at closer range. Some practitioners have studied their field for several years, have much experience and, accordingly, know their limits and do not promise quick fixes. Most forms of CAM share certain features. First, most if not all fall within the realm of private medicine, i.e. health care plans do not cover the expense. Meetings are usually scheduled for one hour duration, although occasionally they may be longer or shorter, and interruptions are rare. In contrast, visits with doctors are usually much shorter and more commonly interrupted. Second, most if not all practitioners have spent quite some effort and time on self-exploration, have been working on their own psychological baggage and know the importance of guiding their patients to do the same. Finally, each practitioner has a special mode of therapy for which success they quote mostly anecdotal evidence, either from their own teachers and/or literature or their personal experience. The patients, on the other hand, after spending time and money are inclined to confirm a beneficial effect. The pragmatic, rational physician in me wishes to see objective proof of efficacy – but I acknowledge that many accepted forms of therapy in modern medicine are also unsubstantiated. Once again, I am willing - and so are most patients - to accept the so-called placebo effect: an improvement of symptoms in spite of absence of proof in randomized, controlled trials.

All this I explained to Mr. Weisman in a few sentences. I then paused and he waited. I sensed he expected more – and I felt relatively comfortable with him to continue. "You and I believe that there is more than meets the eye. With our morning blessings we pray that our eyes are opened with wisdom and that we are released from the bonds that constrict us. With the former we request to understand the meaning of the events of our life; armed with these insights we may attain release from bondage and imprisonment in misconceptions and reflective behavior patterns that harm us and our environment". I paused, looked him in the eye: was he prepared for more? "I firmly believe - but don't have objective evidence from objective research - that many diseases somehow arise from the depths of our souls and, if not taken care of, finally and often symbolically manifest in the physical. Heart attacks, stroke and cancer are all physical diseases that can be measured by imaging techniques and blood tests. However, they may all be the final result of internal processes. Most modern physicians may frown at this contention. However, they readily acknowledge that heart disease and stroke are end-organ diseases that are precipitated by obesity, smoking, a sedentary existence and other lifestyle factors. Hence, we can just take this reasoning one step further: there must be underlying factors in the character and soul of a person that make him adopt and cling to overeating, inactivity and smoking in spite of overwhelming evidence that this may likely lead to harm. I believe the same is true for many if not all diseases".

Mr. Weisman was a careful listener. He completely agreed with me; in fact, the famous Rabbi Moses ben Maimon or Maimonides, who lived a thousand years ago and had been an eminent physician to several kings in addition to being an outstanding Torah authority, had maintained the same opinion. The Talmud advices the patient with a headache or similar symptom to study Torah; this suggests that the cure of many if not all symptoms – before crystallization into irreversible physical disease - may be through the study of Torah. He smiled: "This is preventive medicine. I believe your field of interest is infection control through preventive measures". He evidently had done some internet searching. I smiled back: "In the book of Exodus there is a beautiful sentence that confirms that careful observance of the Torah's precepts may prevent all the diseases that the Egyptians suffered from." He quickly quoted: Exodus 15: 26. We were definitely in rapport and I dared to take the next step.

"We are familiar with the Jewish concept that every problem that befalls us should lead to introspection and review of our deeds. We ascribe the fall of the two Holy Temples in Jerusalem to certain inappropriate behavior patterns of the Jewish people over time. History records that the Babylonians and the Romans ruined the two temples, but we view these destructive empires as the unknowing agents in the hands of God – which, however, did not absolve them of deserved punishment. These people too had a free will and could have acted otherwise – and God would have employed other means to carry out His intentions. On Yom Kippur we pray for atonement of our sins, but not through some disease or ordeal. Implicitly we acknowledge that diseases and ordeals of various kinds serve as powerful inducers to introspection, confession and amendment of our thinking, speech and behavior". I knew I had not said much new to Mr. Weisman. However, so far his knowledge had been theoretical and man's perspectives tend to change with actual experience. The last thing I wish to do is precipitate guilt feelings. I definitely don't want to add distress to a patient, who suffers from a vexing physical symptom, by leading him to believe that he is to be blamed for its onset. I referred him to Rabbi Shalom Arush's book "The garden of faith". "If we accept that all good things derive from heaven, why should not those things that look otherwise come from there as well? The worst one could do, facing an ordeal or disease, is blaming oneself: I deserve this - an attitude that paralyzes and traps us in our predicament. We are steeped in the prophetic literature and Midrashim (biblical stories and legends) that purvey the central message that God is not interested in punishment but wishes man to *amend* his ways, to be just in his actions and modest in his behavior. Finally, Mr. Weisman, I don't want to sound judgmental, preaching or condescending. The doctor and his patient are in the same boat: both of us have to learn something from the interaction to educate and advance our souls. Maybe the only real difference between the doctor and the patient is that the former gets paid for his educated efforts, although a deeper understanding makes us realize that if the patient proceeds appropriately he is the one with the greatest personal gain".

Mr. Weisman was handling himself with dignity and elegance. Even his facial features did not reveal adverse feelings. He remained composed and self-possessed. "You know I am familiar with these concepts. However, knowing these ideas in theory is different from "knowing" them in the same way Adam knew Eve, indicating close contact. I have thought about these things, but it is vastly superior to talk about it with someone. Thinking cannot lead one further than several steps. This is of course the idea behind the proven method of Torah study, in teams of two". He paused. He seemed to deliberate whether to proceed with a new idea. After some moments, when it was evident that he had not yet made up his mind I chipped in. "You know, Mr. Weisman, it is very tempting to start from the acute symptom or disease and try to work backwards. I have gone through this with quite some patients. The initial step is relatively easy: you consider your acute symptom or disease manifestations and start by raising free associations. You then attempt to follow these leads back to your personal history – and that is where one often meets a tall wall. The problem is that if our understanding is correct we are dealing with subconscious processes, perhaps following tortuous pathways that eventually manifest in concrete tissue changes. Moreover, similar triggers may lead to various diseases in different people".

If we had not been dealing with a serious condition and suffering I would have actually enjoyed this meeting of minds. Mr. Weisman was evidently a polished and dignified person with great internal refinement and nobility that were the result of much Torah wisdom and soul searching. "So then", he said, "if the direct way of free association is not the quickest route please tell me about the indirect one that leads to the goal". I smiled: Mr. Weisman was referring to a well known Talmudic story about an elderly man who comes to visit Jerusalem of two thousand years ago. Some distance from the surrounding walls the road splits into two. Fortunately, a young boy sits at the crossroads and the old man asks the boy for directions. He is puzzled when the boy asks whether he would like the "short, long" way, or rather the "long, short" way. He shrugs and randomly selects the short, long way. And the boy shows him the short, long way: short it is, and the gate in the wall is readily visible from the crossroad. However, when the newcomer enters the road, it turns quickly impassable due to overgrowing thorn bush. He first attempts to wade his way through but is obliged to return to the boy at the junction. From there the "long, short way" turns out to be a long and winding path that leads without obstruction to the city gate.

"Mr. Weisman, the long, short way in this instance is indeed longer, it is definitely productive, but surprisingly, it does not lead to one and predefined gate in the wall. Rather, wherever you encounter a wall, an aperture tends to open up". The symbolism was not lost on him and he begged me to continue. Before proceeding, I cautioned him that like with all trials there was no guarantee of success up front, in his case complete cure or even improvement of symptoms. Such is the nature of trials: if you rise to the occasion you may possibly succeed and the gain is yours, while if you fear failure and don't make an attempt you already have failed. I told him that from here it would be his turn. The longer way consisted of the patient being actively involved in a process that exhumes old issues, some of which might be buried deep in the subconscious and work on these with various techniques. I often review with my patients a range of options in order to have them involved in the selective process and increase their motivation and involvement. In Mr. Weisman's case I suggested a combination of two modes of treatment, both in addition to those made by the urologist. First, I suggested he see a medical doctor, who was also a superb and experienced practitioner of classical homoeopathy. He asked an informed question: whether there is anything in the super diluted homoeopathic remedies except water. I indicated that I appreciated his question. "You are right, beyond a certain dilution there is indeed only water and no solvent. However, the succussed and highly diluted remedies have unique nano-structures and qualities that have been scientifically proven; their medical efficacy has as yet been shown only in individual patients. According to practitioners of homoeopathy selecting the appropriate remedy is a difficult art. However, if the correct remedy is selected improvement or cure may be rapid. In my view the homoeopathic remedy is like a lubricant – here I paused briefly - on rust-stuck hinges. An additional treatment is often necessary, in the case of the rust-stuck hinges some vigorous moving to-and-fro".

"So what is the second method you recommend?" I mentioned there are various forms of guided imagery, which induce the mind to readily raise relevant personal issues and emotional memories. One of the easiest and quickest methods is the one developed by Brandon Bays, the author of "The Journey". Mr. Weisman could either attend a two-three day seminar with several hundred other participants, as Bays and her colleagues hold several such seminars each year in various countries, including our own. However, I would recommend that he see a therapist with considerable experience with this technique and give it a try for several sessions – as much as both felt productive.

He briefly deliberated before telling me his decision. "I appreciate your time and effort and trust your insight. I believe you will be able to give me some names and phone numbers? My intuition tells me to follow your recommendations, but I must have your reassurance that you remain in the background. If anything comes up I wish you to be my fallback. And after some time and possible events I would like to come and see you anyway". Trust is the basic building block of the patient-doctor relationship, without which no further practical therapy could be implemented or would be possible. Of course I agreed with Mr. Weisman's request: and I wished him all the possible blessings and luck on this new path that would hopefully lead to full medical recovery.

Nine months passed. It was in the month prior to Rosh Hashanah, the Jewish year, when people are actively involved with soul searching and amending their ways and relationships that I found a recorded message from Mr. Weisman on my answering machine. Much had happened, was there any chance I could see him before the Holidays? When he walked in I was again impressed with his dignified appearance. I wondered whether there was a greater depth of thoughtfulness, tolerance and wisdom in his face – or whether I was simply fantasizing.

"So how have you been, Mr. Weisman and how are you doing?" He smiled, somewhat embarrassed. "I have had a turbulent time - and I guess I blamed you for it many times, especially during sleepless nights. This is the immediate reason I wanted to come to ask your forgiveness". I nodded: there had been nothing he had to be forgiven for, but if requested I would grant it. He silently acknowledged and continued: "You know, I have studied Kabala since I turned forty, but the experiences and insights of the last year have lent my understanding and knowledge a depth I had not attained before. So, I also wish to express my sincere gratitude for opening up avenues leading to gates I did not exist". Both of us knew the interruption I needed to make: First, it had been God who had given him a symptom to work with; at most I had been a guardian who had shown him the way. Second, his new insight confirmed that even events that we initially perceive as the very opposite of good are essentially beneficial. Mr. Weisman evidently had lived through his ordeal and reached a higher level of existence. There was something else: he felt he needed to reassess what had happened before taking the next steps. As I had been the person showing him this direction he would like to have my permission to do this review with me - rather than confide in someone new. "This does not have to take too much time, less than one hour should suffice…"

He started: "I first need to give you a brief account of my life, not unlike I told the homoeopathic doctor and the Journey therapist you sent me too". The Torah starts with "In the beginning" and continues with the story of creation. Every person's life story is one of creation, with something growing out of nothing, a true miracle. What would Mr. Weisman chose to be the beginning of his story? These choices reflect a very deep level of the soul and an individual's perception of the world and oneself.

"My ancestors are from Israel", he started. I saw he was going backwards in time to the second Temple period. Following the Bar Cochbah uprising (132-135 CE) against the tyrannical Roman rule and the terrible destruction they inflicted on our country his ancestors had immigrated to Eastern Europe – and eventually settled in Hungary. His father was born in 1912 in a small town in central Hungary, attended a cheder (religious primary school) and yeshiva, married and had three children before the war. He provided for his family with a small grocery store and his free time he spent on Torah studies. In the Holocaust the entire Jewish community of his town was massacred, his father was one of the few survivors. He had miraculously lived through Auschwitz and numerous deathtraps. Only his deep faith in God had sustained him. The Torah twice describes the disasters, which would and did befall the Jewish people if they fail to follow God's precepts. His father's Bar Mitswah reading had included the first of these two readings and, significantly his own the second of these. At the time, when his grandfather prepared his father for the special day, they had spent a great deal of time on the legal as well as moral meanings of the described curses. His own father had done the same for him too. His father had been a real Hassid: he lived the law and its significance in the very fibers of his body. He had returned from the war weighing 28 kg, ill with tuberculosis and typhus and his entire family had been wiped out: wife and children, parents, siblings and their families. Nonetheless, Mr. Weisman had never heard a word of anger or frustration from his father's lips. After the war his father left Europe on a convoy of refugees organized by Israeli agents, but the rickety boat with its several hundred passengers never reached Israeli shores. It was forcibly intercepted by a British warship and rerouted to Cyprus. His father met his second wife, Mr. Weisman's mother in a refugee camp in Cyprus, where the British incarcerated the pitiful remnants of European Jewry who had not been able to make it past their blockade of Palestine. Although conditions were awful, they were an improvement compared with those of the death camps. Mr. Weisman's mother also came from a Hungarian village; she and a younger sister were the sole survivors of their extended families. Mr. Weisman's mother had been in an experimentation camp run by an infamous Nazi doctor, whose name he would not mention. Once, on Holocaust Remembrance day she was interviewed by a Holocaust museum representative. Mr. Weisman had not been present and his mother refused that the transcript be made public prior to her death. She had cooperated so as to have a written account available of the inhuman actions German doctors had perpetrated on their Jewish victims. One sentence had kept reverberating through her mind throughout these years and helped keep her sane. "This is how people deteriorate when there is no fear of God", the very sentence Abraham had said when he was forced to live with the Philistines and feared they would murder him in order to take his beautiful wife. Mr. Weisman's mother had not been married before the war and she was somewhat younger than his father. Mr. Weisman's oldest brother had been born in Cyprus, his sister was born in nascent Israel and so was he himself, the youngest in 1950.

In spite of the terrible shadow of the war, Mr. Weisman had felt he had had a normal youth. The war was never mentioned at home, although from a young age he was aware he did not have grandparents or relatives because they all had perished in the

Nazi death camps. Religious life and Torah study were the very focus of their lives. They belonged to a closely knit community of ultra-religious people, all of whom were war survivors and were busy piecing their lives together again. The Rebbe played a focal role in the spiritual, moral and even physical resurrection of the community. Mr. Weisman's father had set up a small grocery with a neighbor and this had grown into a large store. In his spare time he went to the synagogue, where the young Mr. Weisman would find his father meditating or dozing. Once, when his father interrogated him, always benevolently, about his Talmud studies and progress, he had had the impudence to ask what Talmud tractate his father was studying. His father had smiled patiently and said he was not able to concentrate any longer, his thoughts would wander. Therefore, upon the Rebbe's advice, he spent much time praying and occasionally listened to Kabala lessons. During the early nineteen fifties his parents received some retribution money; they never wished to use it for themselves, but his father opened saving accounts for his three children to be transferred on the occasion of their marriages.

Mr. Weisman married in his early twenties. As usual in his community he continued studying in the yeshiva for more than a year until his first child was born. He subsequently needed to provide for his family. The sum his parents had saved had grown substantially over the years and it could be used to start a small business. His father stimulated him to consult with the Rebbe, who suggested he set up a laundry, where large and especially poor families could do their washing for a few coins. At the time, many of such families were unable to afford washing machines – and the business proved to be successful. On the one hand he made his living, while leaving him time for Torah study and simultaneously many people were overtly appreciative to have a public laundry nearby. Although he had always kept the prices very low, the business had grown into affiliates in other neighborhoods and other towns.

Mr. Weisman paused. He looked at me as if to make sure I had been listening, but he was evidently reviewing the story for himself. Although Mr. Weisman's life was cast in the shadow of the holocaust, his family had evidently adjusted admirably, especially in view of the parents' terribly experiences. He remained silent somewhat longer, so I dared to ask: What about your own family? Were there any particular business experiences? And how did and do you feel about the Holocaust? He looked quizzically at me: "Have you been in contact with the homoeopath or my therapist?" Of course I had not. But they had evidently asked similar questions.

Indeed, he continued, he had always thought he had enjoyed a normal youth. Most people evidently think so, because they accustomed to their parental home and don't know anything different. The processes of the last few months had made him aware of other feelings. For the first time he had realized the meaning of the words – You resurrect the dead - said before the second blessing in the Standing prayer, recounted three times daily. He now knew that those "dead" also symbolized the dead feelings within a person and these could be miraculously resurrected. "I do not know what has caused the changes in me: the symptom, which has hit me in such a personal and sensitive place; the homoeopathic interview and remedy, or the twelve "journeys" I have made with this therapist. It does not matter". When answering the three questions I had asked as well as his other two caregivers, strong emotions surfaced which had greatly surprised him, but him only. "Please let me continue".

My wife Ornah is also the descendant of Holocaust survivors. Her parents were from Poland and both had been sole survivors of their respective families. Her father had been among the Sobibor camp rebels, who had successfully fled and lived in the forests until the Russian liberation. Ornah's mother had been in Auschwitz and actually knew his mother in that inferno. Her parents had met in Israel after the war of independence, married and Ornah was their only daughter. Ornah's parents had been depressed and dysfunctional throughout her youth and Ornah had often served as her parents' parent: taking them to the doctor, cooking, cleaning the house and talking to the social worker. Ornah had studied social work in a religious college and had worked with Holocaust survivors before their marriage. Mr. Weisman paused, to reflect. "Especially after what had happened, we felt it was our double duty and mitswah to raise a large family. We were confident in ourselves and in God that we had the strength. We have eight children, four of each gender; except the last one all are safely married, thank God, with good partners, observe the Torah and its precepts and manage financially. Our last daughter has Down syndrome. My wife, bless her, has always been a wonderful woman of valor, the central axis of our home, simultaneously taking care of her parents until they passed away. However, when our daughter Becky was born, she crashed. She could not handle another disabled person in her family. Becky is actually a loveable girl, who attends special classes and functions quite well".

Initially, Mr. Weisman had tried to manage the home with his older daughters, but when the latter married, he had to apply to the Rebbe and the community for some assistance. He had learned that giving is so much easier and more pleasant than receiving. He had learned from the Prophet Hosea's tragic life story. Hosea's wife had left him for various lovers and eventually found herself in the gutter. Throughout his ordeal Hosea kept following his wife at a distance, hoping for a change in her behavior and eventually brought her back to his home: not as his wife, but as a wayward family member to be cared for until she would amend her ways. Throughout this personal tragedy Hosea gradually received a wondrous insight: his wife's unfaithful behavior to her loving husband had been like sections of the Jewish people regarding their God. Moreover, quite likely God had made Hosea chose an unfaithful spouse in *order* to let him know how God "felt" about Israel's behavior. This proved the setting for Hosea's prophesies and preaching, exhorting the Jews to amend their ways, be just and tolerant towards their fellow men. Mr. Weisman should have learnt from his wife's depression and Becky's condition that God wanted to purvey him a personal message. A message he should have listened to and worked with, adapting his life accordingly; instead, he attempted to continue with their regular lives which proved increasingly difficult. He had become irritable and inexplicably had quarreled with a subcontractor company servicing his drying machines. The latter had filed a lawsuit against him, which turned out to be a protracted, frustrating and expensive affair. The problem with his sexual function had been the last event. In retrospect he knew that the traffic sign's green light had been flashing and his Peyronie's disease served as yellow light. He hoped that there would not follow a red light. He knew: here it would *have* to stop. Here he himself would have to stop.

Mr. Weisman did not know what homoeopathic remedy he had received and what part it had played in the subsequent roller-coaster he had been and still was in. He had greatly appreciated the detailed interview. The "journeys", on the other had been real eye openers. During the first three he had encountered a silent white fury raging in his soul. Its source, it surmised and not surprisingly was the tremendous suffering that had been inflicted on his parents, ancestors and countless generous of Jews. The fury raged and raged for about three months, and his therapist let him be and stay with his fury until it had burnt out. The next two or three journeys had been spent on variations of his anger at not being able to affect changes when and for whom it really counted. He had not been able to amend his father's suffering and inability to concentrate, evidently distracted by memories of his first family and wartime experiences. He had not been able to alleviate his in-laws' disability and depression. He had not been able to prevent his daughter's Down syndrome, although that was medically possible, nor had he been able to alleviate or cure his wife's depression. Finally, he had been unable to prevent a troublesome and expensive business dispute. He appeared exhausted and flustered.

It was clear Mr. Weisman had been busy during the last nine months with a big clean-out of submerged emotional burdens. I quietly acknowledged his efforts and progress. We were evidently not done, but we ran out of time. If he wished we could make another appointment for another time, perhaps six weeks hence after the holiday season? After he left I made a quick summary of his story, finishing up with some questions. First, how was his wife's health and what was the quality of his marital relationship? Second, did Mr. Weisman have any insights regarding his business conflict? Third, what was the state of his Peyronie's disease?

Two months later, exactly on the appointed hour Mr. Weisman walked in. We shook hands and he started immediately: "I have been looking forward to see you and to complete the review we started before the Holidays. And I am glad we then did not have time to finish up". It appeared he had made notes of our last meeting, as of all previous meetings, including those with the homoeopathic doctor and journey therapist. While making those notes he realized he had avoided some of my questions, regarding his wife and his business lawsuit. He had spent another sleepless night on the latter issue, prayed on it and then made up his mind. He called his lawyer to inform that he wished to settle the lawsuit out of court – even if this turned out more expensive. He then called his opponent, the owner of the company servicing his laundry machines. He informed the latter that the dispute was his, Mr. Weisman's fault and that he wished to apologize for his behavior and suggested to repeat it in public. Moreover, he would fully compensate him for the damage and bad name it might have given him. His former opponent politely thanked him and said he would think about it and consult with his own lawyer. One week before Rosh Hashanah they had met with their lawyers. Once again Mr. Weisman had apologized, ascribed his misbehavior to personal stresses, which explained but absolutely did not justify his ill-tempered demeanor and actions. The final cost had been less than his lawyer had warned him about. He felt great relief to have solved this issue.

I knew Mr. Weisman did not need or wish for my approval. My facial expression and body language had to suffice to convey my appreciation for his moral and practical behavior. Would he continue, or would I need to prompt him? After a few seconds of hesitation he continued. "There remains one major issue: the relationship with my wife. You know, I was raised to honor my wife and meet her needs and those of the family. We never talked much, except regarding the many practical issues of the family. After you diagnosed my PD and sent me on my personal journeys of healing and self recovery I became quite despondent. I had usually made a point of it being pleasant and dignified in my talking and behavior – until matters deteriorated when our last daughter was born and Ornah turned depressive. In retrospect, I believe my behavior was far from rectified, not only in my business dealings but also at home. Several months into the journeys, while fury and anger were keeping me awake at night, I asked Ornah permission to share with her what I was experiencing. She initially was circumspect, but she appreciated my taking care of my PD and therefore agreed. I did not want to tire her so kept my account quite brief". He smiled derisorily: "You wouldn't know it but I actually am able to be brief". It appeared his wife had absorbed his account like a dry flowerpot absorbs water. He shared with her his feelings of being inadequate towards her and Becky, towards people in his business dealings, and towards Heaven. He now knew that deep down he had been furious all the time, but never knew it and that anger had fueled a lot of his language and behavior. He wanted to apologize to her and requested her feedback to be his "helper against himself" to become a more refined and improved husband.

It appeared Mr. Weisman's wife had been dumb stuck, but only for a minute. She had smiled, her face shining with a happiness he had not seen in a long time. She had loved the sharing of his innermost feelings and the closeness that that created. She subsequently asked his permission to share some of her feelings. Mr. Weisman felt anxious: would he be able to handle the emotions of a woman? It appeared he did not have to handle anything; his wife just wished him to listen. She told him about *her* feelings of inadequacy; first, regarding her own parents, whom she had not been able to help sufficiently in her own view. Second, regarding Becky's Down syndrome – because she too had been informed about the testing of amniotic fluid for the presence of Down syndrome, but she had dismissed the doctor's suggestion out of hand. Actually, his wife loved Becky, but Ornah felt that her husband had not been able to handle Becky's birth and ever since he had been even more reserved and withdrawn emotionally than before. Finally, both of them had been raised regarding a minimal sharing of feelings, and ever since she had become depressed she felt she needed her husband's emotional strength and personal closeness more than ever, and she felt even worse because of this need. Both had greatly enjoyed their newly found emotional intimacy, but were not sure how to proceed. In their social setting people did not go to psychologists – and they already had tasted a bit of modern psychiatry when Ornah first turned depressive. Anti-depressant medications had only worsened her condition and she had discontinued all of it. Did I have any recommendations? He proceeded, in my self-conscious opinion a bit mischievously, whether I was in marriage consultations too?

As usual, I tried to answer in an indirect way. "Mr. Weisman, something has impressed me, which you may have given thought as well. Your family name indicates that you are a white or clean man and your laundry business essentially helps clean – or whiten – peoples' used clothes. The first names of both you (Shneor) and your wife's (Ornah) indicate light, like lightening a dark room or shedding light on unsolved issues". I waited to see whether the symbolism was lost on him. It wasn't: I saw his eyes enlarge and lighten up. "It seems to me that you, as so many in our generation, are second or third generation after huge outrages perpetrated against our ancestors. Rather than rage against it, it is our generation's prime responsibility to work through the huge emotional impact we have inherited. The Torah and its 613 precepts are the pre-eminent tools we have received to cope with that huge challenge. However, rather than "whitewash" the dirt or shuffle it under the carpet, we should expose it to full light, examine it, and remove the awful stings. Properly done, we can actually transform our past weakness into our future strength." I was referring to a profound Jewish concept, which holds that any man's past sins, upon gained insight, confession and amendment of ways may lead to a re-found direction of genuine purpose and Self. In my last words there had also been a buried pun, which like anything else he did not fail to pick up.

He was evidently touched, briefly touched his eyes. "Thank you for empowering me, emotionally, spiritually and physically", he said. "I have never mentioned it, but my PD has improved, bending is less severe and there has as yet not been interference with function". I ended the session by giving him the details of a religious husband-wife team, who provided marriage council and support for religious couples. "Please continue with the excellent work you have been doing with yourself and your wife. It seems you are firmly on the road of personal salvation".

Chapter 15: A case of marital conflict and distress

Marriage and its multiple complications have fascinated me since my own wedding, with its subsequent ups and downs and ups. With time and experience I grew in practice and theory. During my youth in the 1950s and 1960s divorce was rare. I vividly remember when I was fifteen and met a nice girl, who informed me that it would not be worth my while to date her because her parents were divorced. I was astounded: what would her parents' situation have to do with our relationship? Since then I have become less innocent: for a starter, children of divorced patients have a greater propensity to break up their own relationships. I am distressed by the epidemic of divorce plaguing western societies, the significant toll divorce extracts from the couples and misery it visits upon their children often for life. I do not know the reason for my interest with marriage and especially for my distress when couples in my vicinity fight and break up. Over time I have read multiple books on the topic of marriage and gained much from each, but only after delving into Jewish wisdom did a deeper level of understanding of the workings of the human soul and couple dynamics open up. During conversations with the medical and nursing staff in our hospital the topic of marriage and associated complications occasionally comes up, at which times I refrain from joining the usual, superficial jokes and prefer to make a constructive remark. This over time has led various physicians and nurses and other personnel to ask for my time and pour out their hearts. In these situations listening is an art and I always have to fight down my urge to say too much. It is vastly more helpful to say only a few sentences, which exactly hone in on one or two central issues. During the next conversation, if there is such, another central theme can be touched. It takes the mind time to process emotional issues and make changes. I always accentuate the fact that I am a physician, not a marriage counselor and urge them to seek expert guidance.

Elishevah Cohen was a nurse working in the same hospital as I do, but in another department. During my residency days she worked in the emergency department, where I spent many nights, weekends and holidays. The sharing of life-and-death events during these night shifts creates closeness in the medical and nursing teams, although there is rarely time to analyze events or their impacts beyond the immediate professional aspects. At the conclusion of the shifts the team disperses, each going off to his and her home and family. One day, many years after completing my residency, Elishevah called and asked whether for the sake of old days I would be willing to see her in clinic for a personal problem. Hospital based physicians are often requested to take care of the medical problems of the staff and of course I agreed immediately. When she came in I remembered in a flash some bits of her history. She was currently in her mid fifties, an attractive woman who took care of her appearance, but in a modest way. She had emigrated from Morocco by boat as a ten-year old girl with an older sister, a huge adventure at the time. Her parents and other siblings only joined after several years. Although hailing from a traditional family, she has grown up with other children in a secular kibbutz. When her parents arrived, she left the kibbutz to help them settle in a town in the north of the country. As her older sister was already enlisted in the army, Elishevah became the parent of her parents; she was the only one who knew the language and who knew the whereabouts. A classical picture developed: her mother quickly learned Hebrew, socialized and started working in childcare, whereas her father, who had been a businessman and solid provider, had difficulty to acclimatize. Like many unskilled male immigrants, who knew only broken Hebrew he could only find low paying, menial jobs and quickly became depressed. "So Elishevah, what is it that brought you to see me?"

She had a family problem and felt stuck. She remembered some comments I had made about conflict solving at the time we worked together in the emergency department, some twenty five years earlier. The family problem was already present and incubating at that time and accordingly she had been receptive to my comments and remembered these vividly. She had four children, two married daughters, a son in the army, while the youngest, a 17 year old boy was still at home. The problem, I already had this sinking feeling in my gut, was her husband. He was a taxi driver, always angry and over time became more and more abusive. Was there violence? Elisheva shifted her eyes away from me. No, there was no overt violence: it was more verbal abuse, a deluge of street language, expressions of frustration regarding the people he met on the job, politics and the "general condition of the country". She did, however, remember two or three instances when he had actually threatened to slap her in the face. Elishevah had asked her husband Aaron several times to go with her to couple therapy, but he just ridiculed and dismissed her, female baloney. Elishevah had spent much time on personal psychotherapy as well as group therapy and had gained significant personal growth and insight. Many years ago she had decided that if her husband did not change for the better she would get a divorce when her youngest son turned eighteen and joined the army, which would be pretty soon. She wished to end her marriage in the least messy way possible and would like to enlist my help.

I was astounded. "Elishevah", I said, "I am a physician, not a marriage counselor and I am definitely not an undertaker who helps bury marriages". She knew as much. Nonetheless, she wished to build on the fact that I had once taken care of her husband and that he had expressed much respect for me at the time and later when the issue of doctor's commitment and expertise came up. I had forgotten, but indeed, Aaron's clinic file showed that I had seen him twice ten years earlier because of acute prostatitis, once in the urology department and then once in the out-patient clinic. Did Aaron know that she wished to get a divorce? They had been several times on the brink of filing for divorce, but each time it had been Aaron who shrank back and promised to improve. I wondered aloud, whether Elishevah had been able to give Aaron adequate expression of her inability to put up with his abusive language and behavior. She actually felt she had done so. And did he make good on his word? Each time he kept his temper for several days until he returned to his usual repertoire. To me it seemed that during one of those crises times Elishevah needed to extract a promise from her husband to enter anger management therapy or couple counseling. She had tried once or twice, because she too felt encouraged that Aaron evidently did not want to split up and therefore should have been more inclined to do something for it. Possibly he was just manipulating her? I agreed to see Aaron once and then would decide to have another meeting with her alone or with both.

During the next several days I had severe misgivings: why had I agreed to this mission? Was it pride, that I would be able to prevent this divorce? Was it perhaps the 15 year adolescent inside, who tried to bring together the divorced parents of his girlfriend? The level headed physician inside reasoned that I would try to convince this man to seek anger management or couple therapy and even if unsuccessful I would refuse to become the surrogate therapist. Perhaps I should call Elishevah and cancel the appointment? Bringing peace between a man and his wife is considered a great *mitswah* (biblical command), a very good deed. However, Elishevah asked me to help her to end their marriage amiably. I decided to call a well known rabbi, an expert in marriage counseling and presented my dilemma. He did not have any qualms: first, if this woman had come to me, intuitively knowing my dislike of divorce, there was hope that she might be amenable to another attempt to salvage their marriage. Second, if the husband had expressed respect for me as physician he might be receptive of my suggestions to seek professional assistance. Finally, he would be willing to talk with me afterwards and provide further guidance.

Aaron walked in exactly on time. He was a thin, middle height man with the wrinkled red-bluish face of a long standing smoker. When we shook hands, I smelt the cigarette smoke on his clothes. "How have you been doing, Mr. Cohen, since we last met ten years ago?" I felt that was a good starting point and he immediately hooked on. After all, the problem then had been medical and physical, which is always much easier for men to refer to than emotional issues. Subsequently, the reason for his visit came up. Aaron said his wife wished him to see me to get him into agreeing to a divorce. At least the issue was clear, no need for circumspect use of words. "And how do you feel about divorce?" It appeared Aaron had given much thought to the issue of marriage and divorce. He felt their marriage was a reasonably successful one, both partners meeting each other's needs most of the time, although not always. "But who does? And which couple doesn't have occasional altercations?" They had married off two daughters, provided for their weddings and supported the young families as much as possible. They had saved for their sons' education and future marriages. They had some friends with whom they occasionally met. They continued to occasionally have sexual relations, which he knew not all of his married friends did. Over time, Elishevah had shared with him her frustrations about the quality of their marriage and had brought up the matter of divorce. It puzzled him; he thought that middle aged women were much more jealous of their marriages, while men of such age were more inclined to look at younger women. He rarely did: he knew his wife was not perfect and he was happy about that. Would she otherwise put up with his insufficiencies?

Aaron appeared much more emotionally developed and self-aware than Elishevah's introduction had made clear. It gave hope and also a growing sense of expectation. I wondered what he felt were his insufficiencies, at least as far as he had learned from his wife. "Oh, I have an Iraqi temperament. I am an emotional type. I don't hide my emotions. If people make me angry, I flare up, which upsets Elishevah. But that is not a reason for divorce. Moreover, it often seems to me that she actually provokes me on purpose. From time to time she brings up the topic of my job. I am a taxi driver. For ten years I was a salaried driver until I saved enough to own my own taxi. Nonetheless, Elishevah continues to accentuate that I am just a chain-smoking, foul-mouthed taxi-driver, while she is a registered nurse. She does not show much respect for me. Quite likely I don't deserve much respect. I am, after all, only a taxi driver, without college degree. However, I worked myself up after growing up in a shanty town of new immigrants. I have noticed that quite predictably I become verbally angry whenever she starts mouthing my job and its frustrations. And believe me it is aggravating to be on the road for twelve hours a day in a city which grows more congested by the day, serving people who become more demanding and less polite by the day. People don't show much respect today. In my youth that was different".

The eminent psychologist Carl Jung described the shadow phenomenon. Each person carries aspects of his individuality which are outside of his own view, suppressed elements, which he himself prefers not to see, but which the close environment easily recognizes. The two short talks with Elishevah and Aaron showed readily accessible issues of importance in their marriage; first, the issue of disparate professional development and, second, its relative importance for each. Moreover, there seemed to be a fit-in pattern: for subconscious reasons they would find themselves time and again in the same fight, unable to prevent or ameliorate its bitterness. After thanking Aaron for his willingness to share, I asked him to tell me a bit about his youth and background. He chose to start far back in history. According to the family tradition, his ancestors had been forcibly moved to ancient Babylon after the destruction of the first Temple by king Nebuchadnezzar at 585 BC. There had been famous yeshivas in Babylon and Aaron knew, or imagined that some of his ancestors had been famous sages, perhaps contributing to the Talmudic literature. Both his maternal and paternal great-grandfathers had been rabbis, but the subsequent generations of his grandparents and parents had become merchants, evidently because of the worsening economic conditions in Arab countries after the beginning of the twentieth century. His father had owned a spice store in down town Bagdad, a well-to-do citizen who in his free time supported the local orphanage and he had served in the local synagogue as secretary of the community. After the war of Israeli independence in 1948, the Iraqi government, whose defeated army had participated in the hostilities, staged small scale pogroms and raids on the local Jewish population. Several hundred thousand Jews, who traced back their ancestry in Iraq for twenty five hundred years were forced to flee, leaving all their possessions behind. Aaron himself had been two years old when the family arrived in the young Israeli state, with nothing save the clothes on their back. They had lived for two years in a tent camp and another two years in a shantytown before moving to a two room apartment in a development town on the coast. In Iraq, his mother had always taken care of the seven children, Aaron being the youngest, but the dire economic situation forced her to start working in house cleaning. On the job she quickly picked up workable Hebrew. His father, on the other hand, had been near sixty when they moved; from a successful, middle aged gentleman, who occupied various respectful social functions, he suddenly felt useless and a burden for his family. He never found a job, remained at home except for going to the local synagogue which provided some structure and comfort. He did not complain but made a point of it to talk and behave respectable. Aaron's father died the day after his bar mitswah from a heart attack; vividly he remembered his father's speech at the celebration, telling him to be a good, honorable citizen, to honor his fellow men, to refrain from lying and cheating, and above all to cherish his future wife and family. Aaron had tears in his eyes when he concluded his story, although he tried to hide them while blowing his nose.

I am always fascinated when patients share their life stories. Quite often there is an apparent association between life's turns and medical, psychological and social events. Aaron and Elishevah shared a similar background; although hailing from different countries, their fathers had been middle class businessmen, amply providing for their families before historical events forced them to leave everything and start from scratch in nascent Israel. Their mothers had adjusted quickly, learning the language, becoming the providers, while the preeminent position of the father figure withered away. I invited Aaron for another meeting, but before concluding our meeting I wished to quote two ancient pieces of wisdom and give him a little homework. First, I reminded him of a "Saying of the Fathers" which appeared in the Oral Law, handed down from Moses throughout the generations and subsequently written down by Rabbi Jehuda Hanassi, about eighteen centuries ago. The book asks: "who is an honorable man?" And it provides the answer: "whoever honors other people". The association with Aaron's father was obvious. Secondly, I wished to refresh his memory regarding the contract, which each Jewish man signs at the marriage ceremony and hands over to his wife. Did Aaron recall its contents? He did not and most likely never knew, because it was in Aramaic and even when "they read it at weddings people usually don't understand it". The contract states that the undersigned husband-to-be undertakes to work to provide for his wife, to honor her, to provide for food, clothes and jewelry and of course help expand the family. I accentuated: after working to support your family, the second obligation is honoring your wife. And according to the "Sayings of the Fathers" once the husband honors his wife, honor of necessity becomes mutual… Finally, regarding the "homework" I asked him to take out the regular prayer book, which he probably had on a shelf, or else go to the local synagogue, and read the letter with instructions which another father had given to his son. Nachmanides, Rabbi Moshe ben Nachman, had written this letter to his son about one thousand years ago. The letter is written in readily accessible Hebrew and appears just before the afternoon prayers in all Sephardic prayer books. We would start our next meeting with Aaron's insights regarding that letter.

On purpose I had scheduled the next meeting two weeks hence. Each needed time to digest the first meeting. Aaron came in with a bashful, boyish smile, almost as if caught at a minor mischief by a teacher at school. After our meeting he had remained in the clinic's waiting room and had written highlights of the visit in his pocketbook. He did not recall having had an hour of such deep personal significance ever since his father's speech at his *bar mitswah*. He had never told anyone his life's story and early childhood difficulties. He had never fully realized the economic, personal and emotional price his parents and countless immigrants had paid in the social upheaval following the rebirth of Israel as well as their impact on the children. In the past two weeks he had thought much and discussed with Elishevah his new insight regarding their common background, with displaced fathers, and mothers who had become the heads of their respective families. He had been shaken by the understanding that it was not Elishevah who did not honor her husband, but rather he, Aaron, who did not honor himself. He concluded his monologue by reporting on his assignment, the letter by Nachmanides to his son. Once again the bashful, boyish smile appeared on his face. He had read it over and again, every single day since our meeting. In the letter the famous rabbi urged his son to "always speak kindly and relaxed to everyone. Doing so, he would rescue himself from anger, which is a very bad characteristic that creates hell on earth. After preventing anger, one should conjure up the trait of humility and ponder where the soul originates and whence it is destined to go. Pride leads a person to feel elevated above his fellow men; rather, man should consider himself to stand before the King, which inculcates a feeling of inferiority and inadequacy". This is definitely the letter of an old and wise man to his more impetuous young son, but its precise and modern language and carefully built arguments have kept it fresh and pertinent up to the present day. Aaron felt it could have been written for him.

"Why", I asked Aaron, "do you feel this letter could have been written for you?" His answer was quick and to the point: "because I am angry a great deal of the time. At my customers, who stop me at the most impossible and dangerous intersections; at the other drivers and pedestrians, who make traffic mistakes that could lead to disasters. It is an instinctive anger that erupts all the time". But I wondered why Aaron was angry with his wife. This question brought a frown of introspection on his brow. After a minute or so he said slowly that there are several levels of answering my question: first, he was in the habit of easily becoming angry and, accordingly, whenever something disruptive came up his response was one of anger. He did not know that anger was such a bad trait, how to prevent it from erupting and never had learned the need or method to defuse it. Second, he usually did not express his anger and frustrations at his clients, mostly saved that for his wife in the belief that she could handle that, although he now realized that this was quite unfair. Third, and this was his most important point, perhaps they were re-enacting the play of their respective parents. Aaron slowly formulated his thoughts. Perhaps Elishevah had chosen him, with his lack of higher education, in order to copy her own mother's prominent position at home after the immigration to Israel. Perhaps he himself had chosen Elishevah with her higher education and stronger position, because he identified with his own father, in order to express anger for both himself and his father at the unfairness of it all. And an even deeper idea occurred to him: perhaps Elishevah continued to provoke him, *in order* to have him grow and become the respected, honorable person his father had been, even after he became dethroned as head of the family. Aaron was, after all, the descendant of a long line of rabbis, who could date their ancestry back to the first high Priest, Aaron, Moses brother. Yes, indeed, he was called after the first High Priest. He suddenly remembered that his father had referred to that too in his *bar mitswah* speech, the day before he died. Perhaps he, Aaron had intuitively shied away from that lofty ideal. Perhaps Elishevah was the agent who consciously or not was helping him to get to his senses?

Silently I had watched Aaron, while he delved and dug into deep layers of his soul. I was moved and impressed. This so-called uneducated, chain smoking taxi driver had great capacity for introspection and emotional production. Once again I myself recognized that stereotyping people was superficial, while staying open minded and open hearted could lead to more opening of minds and hearts and increasing closeness between people. Aaron was evidently moved by himself, his head facing down, watching his hands. After several minutes he looked up, our eyes meeting. "This", he said after he broke the silence, "is a moment of holiness". He needed to retain his newly found ideas and asked my permission to jot these down quickly.

After Aaron collected himself, I said I would like to finish this memorable meeting by making a connection, with his permission, between the ideas he expressed and a relevant sentence in the Biblical story of creation. After the creation of man God said: "it is not good for the man to be alone. I will make him a counterpart (literally, a helper against him)" (Genesis 2: 18). The first part of the sentence does not state that it is good to be together: it states that loneliness is not good. God created the "hardware", the woman so that Adam would not be alone. However, in order that their being together actually would be beneficial, the man and his wife actually have to produce and maintain the "software" of their relationship. Although unstated, God clearly invited man to be a participant in His creation. The second part of the sentence explains how this relationship should work. The woman was intended to be his helper, occupying a contra or opposite position. True and proper help consists of being faithful to a higher ideal rather than being a yes-man or yes-woman. The woman is man's faithful companion when she helps the development and emergence of the very best within her husband, while simultaneously helping him expose and conquer his shadow underside.

Two weeks later Elishevah called. She and Aaron had recently had some interesting conversations at home. His behavior was changing: he repeatedly expressed his appreciation for all that she had done and continued to do for him and their children, including bearing up with his mood and behavior, which, he acknowledged was not always optimal. He had started to go to evening services in the synagogue in their neighborhood, usually followed by a lecture by the local rabbi. She was not fully prepared for this religious change and wondered where this would lead to. I challenged her: was she by chance concerned that if Aaron turned more traditional and better behaved that consequently the case for divorce would dissipate? A several second silence at the other end indicated that I had struck a tender cord. In order to help her recollect, I suggested that there was perhaps an additional and positive element to her concern. Maybe Aaron's turn to traditional habits and values had some appeal to her too, because of their similar backgrounds, but the associated changes in outward and spiritual lifestyle felt perhaps threatening? I vividly remembered what happened next: she started crying, a helpless cry, but simultaneously one of relief, as if a longstanding obstruction had finally given way. "Please forgive me. I need to go. I'll think about what you said".

During the next day or two I was concerned what I might have precipitated and some wild fantasies crossed my mind. I was happily relieved when I found a message from Elishevah in my answering machine: they had agreed to go to couple therapy.

Doctors very often have emotionally charged interactions with their patients. The latter may respond in different ways, ranging from anger and resistance to sincere appreciation and gratefulness. Occasionally, like in the case at hand, patients cut all contact abruptly and completely, which makes this physician wonder where he went wrong, or whether he had said or did the wrong thing. Could I have said or done something more sophisticated or more beneficial? Perhaps the patients are embarrassed because of something they did or said? As there are not many such cases, I may initiate some contact after some time. In the Cohen's case, I waited some eight months, alternating between feelings of inadequacy regarding my management of the situation and hope that something positive was developing. They clearly did not need me or even inform how they were doing. Did I need their dependency, their appreciation? I sent them a card on the occasion of Rosh Hashanah, the Jewish New Year, wishing them the usual blessings for a good and healthy and prosperous year. Upon which Elishevah called: "Could we come together for the follow up visit which we had intended and never took place?"

They were evidently relaxed. Elishevah wore a dress, while I remember she used to wear jeans. The major chance was that of Aaron: he wore a small skullcap, had gained weight while his jeans had made place for regular pants. More significant was his face: the frustrated, angry look had made room for a quiet, boyish smile. We looked at each other and I wondered who would start. After half a minute or so of silence, a long time in such a situation, Elishevah looked at Aaron, who nodded and she then started by apologizing for having broken of all contact. She had felt absolutely in shock after our last phone call and she had cried for hours. When Aaron got home, Elishevah informed her about the upsetting call. Rather than becoming angry, he had quietly prepared them a cup of tea and then invited her to describe her feelings. Just tell, just tell and he would just listen, and that response by itself caused her to start crying again. They had been exhausted when they finally went to bed, but slept like babies. The next day Aaron asked her whether she was still willing to go to couple therapy after he had turned down her past requests. Since then much had happened. Elishevah had agreed to Aaron's request, provided that he would move out of the house for some time. Aaron had not protested: he had lived with one of his sisters for about six weeks before his wife agreed to his return. They went and still were at couple therapy. Several months ago Elishevah had agreed to accompany Aaron to a meeting with his Rabbi. Surprisingly, the latter recommended that she should continue with "just the same good work" she was doing, without religious coercion of any kind. The rabbi mentioned that she was the perfect wife, who incessantly had worked to get her husband become a better person, get in closer contact with his innermost feelings and loose "false self" elements, which every person accrues throughout life, from his parents and society. The rabbi mentioned that Aaron had a secret wish: he would like to sing at the dinner table on Friday nights, Sabbath eve, "A woman of valor", a song of deepest appreciation sung in all traditional homes and which both remembered from their own childhood. Would she agree with that?

Before leaving, Aaron said that he looked at his wife as his savior and to me as his "midwife, who has assisted me to give birth to something precious that had been quietly incubating for a long time". Another analogy that had occurred to him, perhaps less flattering, was that of a blacksmith who sprayed a rust-dissolving spray on a long stuck hinge and then started getting it to move again. Their marriage was definitely on the move. They were working, individually and as a couple. "And by the way, I have cut back on smoking, from two packs a day to one in every other. After a lifetime of being admonished by Elishevah I finally got it: she is not mothering me, she is concerned for my health." Once again he smiled that embarrassed, boyish smile.

I recalled what the marriage counseling Rabbi had told me: "First, before seeing a couple pray that you will serve as an agent of delivery rather than of destruction. Second, carefully remember: try to detect issues of emotional significance in the persons you are working with and directly engage these and, if possible, refer to a relevant idea in the Torah or their own value system. That helps to change the paradigm, casts the misery and anger of the involved person or couple into a much wider, universal frame and often induces them to start working on their issues in a fresh and constructive way. Finally, if the couple succeeds to outgrow their problems it is their achievement and theirs only, while at most you served as faithful middleman. This last note of caution is crucial, because inevitably not all couples will make it, in which case you may start blaming yourself and become depressed. This is simply misplaced pride".

Chapter 16: Suicide: A story of jealousy and ambition.

It was near six o'clock in the evening. It had been a long day: I had been called at four in the morning to the intensive care unit (ICU) to see a patient with bacterial meningitis, a potentially lethal and contagious disease. Right now I was going home, bag in hand, heading for the door of my office. Before I reached it there was a knock, the door opened and the anguished face of a young man looked in. "Could I *please* come in for a moment to talk with you?" He was in such obvious distress and his voice had such a pleading edge that I simply could not refuse. I offered him a chair and we sat down. I had seen his face before, but it took a second before I recognized him. Twelve hours earlier I had seen him walking restlessly in the waiting room of the ICU when I spoke with the relatives of my patient with meningitis. He appeared in his late twenties, black skullcap, white shirt and black trousers; he looked like a scholar with bright eyes and high forehead radiating intelligence. He introduced himself as Raphael Shuchat, the husband of Rivka Shuchat, who had been admitted to the ICU that previous night in critical situation on account of a suicide attempt. In agitated sentences, he gave a brief account of what had happened. His wife had swallowed a box of tricyclic antidepressants and maybe three or four boxes of paracetamol. Raphael himself had found the empty boxes in the bathroom during the night. When he returned to bed he noticed that his wife was breathing very shallow and she would not wake up when he called her. She had been depressive for several months after her last delivery six months earlier. Since about three weeks she received an oral antidepressant from the family doctor and Rivka actually reported recently that she felt somewhat better. Raphael had called an ambulance, who inserted a tube into her stomach and another tube into her trachea to support her respiration because she was barely breathing. In the hospital she was quickly transferred to the ICU for monitoring of electricity problems with her heart, induced by the tricyclic antidepressants. The stomach wash did not reveal residual tablets, a sign these had been swallowed many hours earlier. The doctors gave her activated charcoal through the naso-gastric tube to decrease absorption of the residual tablets. In addition, there was fear for liver damage due to the large dose of paracetamol, for which she received an intravenous antidote. In spite of his grave concern, this young man who spent his entire life in the study of the Torah had grasped the essentials of his wife's critical situation.

While Raphael gave the brief account of what had happened, I opened his wife's medical file in the computer, including her laboratory tests, chest radiogram and electrocardiogram. I also called the resident on call in the ICU and she basically supported Raphael's account. Although Rivka was still intubated and mechanically ventilated and would remain so for another day or two, she was expected to survive. The electricity problems with her heart would probably dissipate once the remnants of the tricyclic antidepressants were secreted from her body. Liver functions would probably get back to normal with completion of the intravenous course of acetylcholecysteine, the antidote for paracetamol. There would hopefully be no residual neurological defects, but time would show. Suicide attempts are unfortunately not so rare, but, if the patients are detected on time, which appeared to be the case in this instance, most survived without sequelae. However, Rivka would definitely need psychiatric care and follow-up; in fact, a psychiatrist had already been consulted. I tried to reassure Raphael along these lines. "Maybe you go home, look after your children, eat and rest. You cannot do anything for your wife while she is still sleeping. Tomorrow she may need you next to her." It also flashed through my mind that once Raphael would go, I could go home too, a somewhat inappropriate thought that would shortly be corrected. He did look relieved that his wife would most likely survive and hopefully without permanent damage. Nonetheless, the aura of anguish was still all over his face, his voice and his body language. He swallowed, his face blushing, then turned grey; he was evidently chewing on something unpalatable. Finally he was able to get it of his heart. "You know", he started in a barely audible voice: "I have brought her to commit suicide". He heaved and sighed deeply, evidently on the verge of bursting into tears.

While I stepped out to get Raphael a cup of water, I briefly called my wife to let her know that I unfortunately could not yet leave hospital. Families of doctors often pay a significant price for their spouses' professional activities. As so often I felt torn between my wife and children and this young, anguished man in my office. I would try to make this interview as brief as possible and invite him back the next day. Raphael's confession had evidently provided some relief. After reciting the appropriate blessing he had some water. He did not need further stimulation. Looking downward to the floor, he recounted in a low voice the events leading up to his wife's suicide attempt. "You know, I come from a family of rabbi's. According to the family's genealogy, an ancestor of mine studied with the famous Vilna Rabbi Eliahu four centuries ago and subsequent generations have almost all been rabbis. I have always attended the best yeshivas, but have never been proud of my accomplishments as I know that my background, education and Heaven have provided me with the gifts of intelligence and good manners. When I turned twenty four, my parents arranged my marriage with Rivka, the daughter of a wealthy family. The only girls I knew at the time were my sisters, so I trusted my parents' wisdom. Actually, when I first met Rivka I recalled the description of Rachel, Jacob's wife in the Torah: "shapely and beautiful". And just as has been described regarding Isaac after he married his Rivka, I too have become greatly attached to my wife and love her very much. She is so kind, shy and such a woman of valor! And in spite of several pregnancies and obstetric problems, she has remained *so* beautiful up till the present day. My problem is that I have become exceedingly jealous at anyone who just glances at her. I am consumed with jealousy during the daytime and it has become the substance of my dreams at night. In the beginning of our marriage it was not so overt. Rivka was a kindergarten teacher and almost only met with other women and girls. However, once she became pregnant she needed to see an obstetrician; I could not bear the thought that another man would touch her, so I begged her to change to a female doctor."

Raphael paused, evidently composing his feelings and thoughts. "The first pregnancy ended with the birth of a severely malformed baby, who remained in the neonatal intensive care for two months until she died. Both of us were very much shaken, but our faith sustained us. Genetic counseling indicated that we are both carriers of an unusual genetic disease. The only option to have healthy children is through pre-implantation genetic diagnosis and in-vitro fertilization. Rivka's ova would be aspirated, I would donate sperm and the doctors would mix these and let the fertilized eggs grow into six or eight cell embryos. Then they would do complicated tests to see which embryo does not carry the bad gene and insert it in Rivka's uterus. After three of such procedures Rivka became pregnant and she gave God bless birth to healthy twins, a boy and a girl, now three years old. One and a half year ago, we again started with the same fertility procedures and, as mentioned, six months ago she gave birth to another healthy boy. However, the doctors and staff in the fertility clinic taking care of us are mostly male – and I have been going crazy with the thought that these people look at and touch Rivka. I know I have been bothering her time and again with my jealousy. She keeps reassuring me that there is absolutely no basis for my jealousy. She is so sweet and innocent and I am absolutely sure that there is no shade of thought in her righteous person about any man other than me. She *is* the "woman of valor" personified. So how come I am obsessed with jealousy??"

I appreciated Raphael's honesty and disclosure. However, I wished to reassure him that Rivka's obstetric history could have been part of her depression; moreover, post-partum depression is quite common. In fact, according to Raphael's account it seemed that she was responding quite nicely to the oral anti-depressants. It is not unheard of that several weeks after starting these medications depressed people start to improve, their lethargy makes way for new-found energy and - before their depression completely subsides – this energy may provide the strength to make a suicide attempt. This is one major reason I resort to anti-depressants only if the depressed person is unable or unwilling to do actual emotional and spiritual work with an appropriate therapist. I believe that the latter route is the most physiologic and effective, although unfortunately many people prefer the passive swallowing of pills. I carefully explained to Raphael that of course he would have to work on his jealousy and defuse it, but it did not seem appropriate that he took himself to blame for his wife's suicide.

He smiled ruefully. "There is something else I haven't told you yet – and I am deeply ashamed of that too. After the birth of our youngest son, Rivka has been to the mikveh (ritual bath) only once and very soon became impure again due to intermittent spotting. The last time she saw spotting was about six days ago; according to the Halachah she was scheduled to go to the mikveh tomorrow night. However, tomorrow we were scheduled to go for the weekend to another city due to a wedding in Rivka's family. Of course there is a mikveh nearby, but we would stay over with multiple family members in a small apartment, not allowing for any intimacy. After abstinence of so many months I more or less begged Rivka to be together before leaving for her family. She resisted very much, a real righteous woman, while I am an impetuous young man, who after all my Torah study still needs to conquer his base instincts and jealousy. In the end I convinced her with an argument I am almost too ashamed to mention." He deliberated, swallowed, but continued: "In the Talmud it says that men ought to be deeply appreciative of their women if only for two reasons". I nodded: I knew what he meant: for saving their men from the sin of wasting seed and for raising the children. He paused, all the time looking at the floor. "She must have taken those tablets soon afterwards, while I, stiff-headed sinner and selfish fool, had fallen asleep".

Carefully and respectfully I absorbed this young man's words. We knew only half an hour, not counting the wordless encounter in the early morning hours of that day and he had already disclosed two most intimate matters from his personal life. First, Raphael suffered from an unexpected and all consuming jealousy regarding his evidently angelic wife. In addition, he had coerced his wife into intimacy before her appropriate ritual immersion. Many years ago I had encountered a suicide attempt made for similar reasons; in that case, the involved woman believed that the inappropriate encounter could lead to birth of a malformed baby and in desperation had tried to take her life. In Rivka's case such fear could not have been her motivation: she took oral contraceptives upon her doctor's advice and with her Rabbi's approval because of their genetic problem. Possibly, just the sheer idea that she had failed to induce her husband to follow the Halachah may have been unbearable to her. Rather than blame him, she must have blamed herself to fulfill her duty and stimulate and strengthen her husband in his religious observance. Religious Jews aim for life on a very high spiritual plane, which is not always easy to attain or maintain, although observance of the Torah's precepts essentially provides the tools and ladder. Even if failure dooms now and then, these dips are considered of temporary nature and of necessity lead to subsequent peaks.

There was not much I could say to console Raphael. Anyway, he would not want to be consoled as he was still very much blaming himself. This young man had spent his entire life in religious study, while I had never attended a yeshiva – so he would likely counter any arguments that I could offer to raise his spirits. After an appropriate silence I expressed my appreciation for his frankness. I muttered something like: "According to our sages there are three proven steps of amending one's ways: repentance, confession and subsequent sweetness, resulting from the profound change one has affected in one's character, behavior and speech. It seems you have made a clean start and you should probably go and consult with your Rabbi." He thanked me for my time and allowing him to express his sorrow and guilt feelings.

On my forty-five minute drive home my thoughts wandered back to the young woman fighting for her life in the ICU, her husband and the psycho-social and religious predicaments which were evidently the trigger for the suicide attempt. I thought about jealousy, and a well-known statement from the Sayings of the Fathers popped up. The Mishnah or Oral Law was received by Moses on Mt. Sinai and transferred throughout the ages until it was finally written down by Rabbi Jehuda Hanassi about eighteen centuries ago. This particular statement is ascribed to Rabbi Eliezer Hakappar and holds that "jealousy, passion and the pursuit of honor shortcut people's lives". Commentators write that jealousy concerns other people's possessions, position or luck; passion concerns physical pleasures; while honor indicates the pursuit of social position and power. All of these shorten people's lives, but also compromise one's peace of mind. Next, my mind wandered to two prime examples of jealousy described in detail in the Bible with their destructive impact. The first example is the story of Cain and Abel, as illustrated elsewhere in this book. For unknown reasons, God accepted Abel's offering of a goat but discarded Cain's offering of agricultural produce. Cain becomes very jealous of his brother, but is warned by God to conquer his passion as sin is imminent. Cain does not heed this warning and the jealousy in his heart leads to action: he murders Abel. Did his jealousy and the resulting action lead to any improvement in his condition, would God subsequently accept his offer? As a result of Cain's uncontrolled passion he receives a double curse: the earth would not yield its produce to him any longer after it had absorbed his brother's blood. In addition, he would have to wander about with a sign on his head warning people not to kill him lest his punishment be shortened.

The other biblical example concerns Joseph, whose brothers were jealous of him because their father Jacob appeared to love him better than his siblings – as Joseph was his youngest son and the son of his best loved wife Rachel, who had died in childbirth. The brothers' jealousy turns into hatred, which led to action: the selling of Joseph into slavery. The biblical story and turning of events are masterful and have been a source of inspiration throughout the ages. The root cause of the Jewish immigration to Egypt and their subsequent enslavement can be traced back to sibling rivalry and jealousy.

I did not doubt that Raphael was very familiar with these stories. He probably had learned many Midrashim (Legends) and scholarly Talmudic explanations regarding these biblical stories. Moreover, I knew that in his Haredy (ultra-orthodox) background much attention and time are spent on the refinement of one's character, such as conquering of anger and pride, the use of clean language and development of modesty. Many books on morality have been written by erudite sages throughout the ages to inculcate these characteristics. I thought about Rabbi Chaim Luzatto's "The Path of the Just" written in Italy several centuries ago. I did not doubt that Raphael had studied these books extensively and of course he knew the prescription to conquer one's base instincts, starting with the love of the Torah's precepts up to the fear of punishment by God. Nonetheless, he still had not been able to conquer his jealousy and passion. I doubted Raphael would return to me for further talk on these issues and even if so I would stick to my recommendation, i.e., that he seek guidance from his rabbi.

Sigmund Freud derived his concept of superego from the notion that throughout early childhood normative people of all cultural backgrounds acquire a kind of internalized policeman, who controls their behavior whether of religious or secular persuasion. The superego is essentially based on the internalized fear for punishment from one's parents as well as a craving for approval from one's social environment – and both are essential tools for survival and success. In religious people there is another formidable, double-edged safeguard against uncontrolled expression of basic instincts: the belief that God knows one's very thoughts and that punishment may follow death into eternity. Nonetheless, throughout the years I have met many people, who were tormented by their superego and religious constraints but nevertheless had been unable to control their passions. Examples of these passions range from the use of unrefined language to sexual misconduct, from emotional abuse to antisocial activities. There is, therefore, need for additional advice and educational measures for these people to help them modify their reflective speech and reflective behavior. In addition, the Torah commands men not only to prevent the *expression* of one's passions, but to actually *vanquish* those passions from one's heart. This command makes us realize that essentially all men need to address their passions in order to prevent their expression, but also their very presence in our hearts. Experience and extensive learning have led to the realization that there is only one recipe to accomplish that object: looking at the monsters in the basement of one's soul, getting at the source of their power and then see these hidden drivers of our thinking, speech and behavior evaporate. Almost invariably people need extensive guidance with this process, as our intuition strongly pushes us into any other direction rather than address our basic fears – and tries to seduce us into fooling ourselves into the belief that these problems will dissipate if ignored.

Rivka Shuchat improved as expected. She was successfully weaned from the mechanical ventilator and extubated after three days. She regained consciousness and there appeared to be no residual neurological damage. After she was transferred to a department of internal medicine for further observation, Dr. Jacobs, the consulting psychiatrist attempted to evaluate the risk for further suicide attempts. However, Rivka appeared uncooperative; she refused to disclose the reason for her suicide attempt and remained despondent. Dr. Jacobs felt that enforced admission to a psychiatric institution was called for until psychiatric medications would lead to clinical improvement of depression and reduced risk for a subsequent suicide attempt. When this decision was discussed with her husband, he appeared very reluctant on account of the associated stigma. He mentioned that he had spoken to me on the first night of his wife's admission and requested that the psychiatrist involve me. When Dr. Jacobs called and stated the purpose of his call, I told him that I had received privileged information from Raphael and needed his approval before further discussing. After Raphael gave his somewhat reluctant agreement, the three of us discussed how to proceed. Raphael and I would try to talk with Rivka and if we were successful in getting her cooperation, Dr. Jacobs would subsequently join us. If unsuccessful, Dr. Jacobs would arrange for the transfer to the psychiatric institution. We had our one chance: careful preparation and prayer for success were definitely called for. I invited Raphael to my room to discuss the upcoming talk with his wife.

I warned Raphael that the three-way meeting with Rivka might not be easy for him. I would use the information he had volunteered in our first meeting. Possibly I would raise other issues that he might interpret as criticism or even condemnation. "Please refrain from doing so: the focus of our meeting is your wife and her benefit. You should be ready with some forbearance, especially after you told me that you feel somehow responsible for at least part of your wife's current condition". I waited for his confirmation and then proceeded. "I know you are steeped in Torah study and have absorbed much of its wisdom. Nonetheless, you have pointed at two of your characteristics that in your own view are deplorable, have negative implications for yourself and your family and deserve rectification. I think it is important that you get a closer handle on those issues before we start talking with Rivka." After a short pause I asked: "I wonder whether you have had a chance to talk with your Rabbi after our first talk". His face and body language readily disclosed he had not. He blushed, his body slouching forward to hide his face. I tried to reassure him. "Don't worry. I am not surprised. People absolutely hate to encounter the bad stuff in their basement. However, the road to Rivka's cure probably involves a continued effort from you too. I am not talking about lip serve, but about a real investment on your part". He indicated that if I was *certain* that this would lead to the desired outcome he of course would contribute his bit. "You know, Raphael, when Abraham went through his ten tribulations he did not know whether he would succeed and he did not know up front what their outcome would be. However, he was "innocent before God": he *knew* that everything came from Heaven and therefore he had to refrain from questioning their fairness or purpose, but readily focus on working through. Abraham believed that all trials came from Heaven and were therefore for man's benefit, even if that benefit appeared elusive at the current time. Raphael, you and your wife are presently experiencing a tremendous challenge. You cannot see the benefit right now, only the suffering. However, when Abraham overcame his tribulations successfully he could look backward with the certainty that God had guided him into attaining a higher level of personal and spiritual maturity. You know I could not possibly promise you a specific outcome. I can, however, pledge to do my best and together we should hope that I serve as a good messenger".

Once again I received proof that reframing of a patient's problem in terms of his system of belief or values was supremely beneficial. The reframing elevates the patient above his immediate suffering and transports him to a higher level even before he has started working on himself. Rather than being pulled down by his suffering, the patient is able to look upward and beyond his immediate distress and start wondering at its meaning. Raphael was completely engaged and we were resonating nicely. Only with this level of agreement could I reasonably expect to have his cooperation with the next step. "Raphael, several days ago you told me that in your feeling the expressions of your jealousy have been painful to Rivka". I waited: was he following? I then continued: "When God refrained from taking Cain's offer, he became very jealous of his brother Abel, whose offer was accepted. The Torah does not state the reason for God's differential approach, although various sages have offered illuminating comments. The instruction we obtain from this story is not an insight regarding the source of jealousy. Rather, the Torah wishes to instruct us that once we feel jealous that we should conquer it, because otherwise it leads to bad action, starting with inappropriate speech and culminating with murder. As you experienced yourself, the fear of punishment is not sufficient to banish strong feelings from one's heart. I suggest we do a little experiment. You close your eyes, take several breaths to relax and then you look at the well of your jealousy. Think about one or two situations when you felt your jealousy most acutely, when it almost prompted you into bad talk or actions. Nod with your head when you have arrived".

It was a simple, but powerful technique. Raphael cooperated. He closed his eyes, I guided him through his deep breaths and he observed that that made him feel good. He remained quiet for several minutes; I then stimulated him in a soft voice: "Jealousy, Raphael, think about a particular bad instance of jealousy". After some time he nodded. I prodded him to stare at it, closely feel and taste it. He blushed. "Now Raphael, what is at the root of that jealousy? What feeds it?" It took perhaps ten seconds, before he whispered: "Feeling inadequate and inferior". I whispered back: "Thank you. Please look at those feelings of inadequacy and inferiority, feel and taste those feelings. Now, what is at the root of that jealousy? What feeds it?" It evidently took a major effort, but he persisted. He finally heaved and whispered: "Utter nothingness. Death." I was impressed at the fast pace with which Raphael had evidently been able to get at the source of his affliction. For several years he had tried to kill the feeling or run away from it, but time and again it had popped up its head and had induced him to speak and behave obsessively. It was an inner force behind his Self that was driving him. Once again I felt deeply privileged to be a doctor, on whom patients rely with their greatest problems and innermost feelings. "Thank you, Raphael for your honesty and willingness to disclose. Please take your time. Take deep breaths. Only after you feel you are ready you may open your eyes". Raphael remained silent for several minutes, evidently emerged in thoughts and feelings that had as yet not been accessible to him.

At least we had privacy: Rivka had a single patient room. Raphael had a chair on one side of her bed, while after introducing myself I sat down on the other side. Rivka looked pale, her face drawn and she stared at her feet. There are two ways of talking with a depressed person. The first consists of presenting actual evidence from that person's life that there is no objective reason to feel depressed. This approach is doomed to fail; the patient knows her own parameters quite well and in spite of these feels awful and depressed. Presenting the "facts" only accentuates the depressed person's misery. The other way is by trying to identify with the patient's feelings of depression. I call this the chicken approach according to a well-know Hassidic fable. In that story, the king of a certain country had one son, the crown prince, who one day appeared to lose his mind. He undressed and hopped nakedly on one leg, all the while kukureeku-ing like a chicken and picking at morsels on the ground. The king was at his wits' end as doctors from all over the empire failed to cure the prince. Finally, a wise old man came around and volunteered to cure the prince. Everyone wondered: how could this sage cure the prince where famous doctors had failed?

Upon everyone's surprise, the sage undressed and joined the prince, who was sitting under a table, busy picking at morsels. The sage also started hopping on one leg and kukureekood like the prince. After some time the prince looked in surprise at the sage, then asked: "who and what are you?" Upon which the sage answered that he was a chicken, just like the prince and he was behaving accordingly. They continued happily together for some time, after which the sage engaged the prince. "You know, the fact that we are chickens does not mean that we cannot wear pants". He put on trousers himself and induced the prince to do so to. After more happy hopping, kukureeku-ing and pickings, the sage observed to the prince that they could be happy chickens to themselves and the entire world, while they wore shirts. Gradually, the sage talked the prince into dressing, getting out from under the table and into adopting normative behavior, while all the while sharing with him the illusion that they were perfect chickens. The parable can be dissected and analyzed in multiple ways. One important layer addresses the uniqueness of every individual, accentuates each person's specialness while seamlessly allowing for the functioning of society.

"Mrs. Shuchat, I know you feel awful." I knew intuitively that I would not call her by her first name. I rarely call my patients by their first name and teach my students and residents to refrain from doing so. This formality helps define the rules of the patient-doctor relationship and fosters mutual respect. However, in a patient much younger than you are one may be easily tempted to flout the rule. I thought this patient would prefer the respect of being called by her family name, because a lack of respect might be the root cause of her depression. Moreover, I felt that this young woman probably felt inadequate in the presence of her husband and another male, a doctor. "I guess that you have felt awful for quite some time and that things slowly have become unbearable to you". Each sentence was pronounced precisely and deliberately, to be followed by a short pause to have her absorb its contents and tone. "Raphael has told me about the two of you and your three children. He has told me that you are his "woman of valor", his faithful "helper against himself", who restively strives to assist him to express the very best towards fellow men and God". Rivka glanced briefly at Raphael as if to ascertain that he indeed had told as much; and perhaps also to make sure that he had meant these things. I was glad at that first acknowledgement of our presence. I continued: "You know, Raphael has told me that he feels inadequate towards you. While you are his guardian good angel he feels that he fails you. He also fails himself, to live up to the high standards that he expects of himself and that he knows that his and your family expect of him too".

Rivka threw a brief glance at me. After looking back at her feet she said in a low, hoarse voice: "Raphael is the perfect angel. I am the failure". She then started to cry, a desolate cry as if on the brink of an abyss. I watched as Raphael handed her a tissue. Overt signs of intimacy between ultra-religious couples are avoided at all cost; I therefore respected this subtle sign as the closest to care for his wife that Raphael might show in public. The gesture was not lost on Rivka: she glanced at him as if to make the most of this sign of care. The silent pantomime between these young people was touching. They were highly gifted, each in her and his own way, evidently cared about each other, but possible did not know how to express their feelings or how to get across to their spouse. On the other hand, they had been primed with the loftiest ideals and felt inadequate when they could not live up to these ideals all the time. I had a sudden intuition. I accosted Raphael.

"In the story of creation, after the story of the snake and the apple, Adam's punishment is to go out in the world and provide for his family. Eve's is to have painful deliveries, while "her passion is for her husband who rules over her". The simple meaning of this verse indicates that the husband earns the money, while his wife cares for the home. There is mutual dependence between a man and his wife, each providing for the needs of the other and both supplement the other. However, the un-rectified man may live with a false sense of pride as "if he had created his own ability" of earning the money that makes the family function. His wife, on the other hand, is acutely aware of her and their children's dependence on her husband. She therefore works hard to please her husband; she thrives on his approval, it provides her with strength to cope with the endless challenges of the children and the home - and she cringes at the slightest word or even tone of criticism. You know, Mrs. Shuchat, it has happened in quite some homes of brilliant yeshiva students that these young men come home and bedazzle their wives with their knowledge of the Talmud. They tend to correct their wives regarding the ways the Torah's precepts should be carried out appropriately. Instead of helping with the household chores they may criticize their wives: that the home is not organized, that the meal is not ready when they come home, that the children are not cared for appropriately. It has driven women to misery, to seek divorce or worse…"

Silently I watched the couple look at each other. I had quoted from a chapter in "The Garden of Peace", a compendium on attaining and retaining peace at home, but also from experience with other couples. My intuition was not misled. Raphael was not his family's provider: according to the prenuptial agreement he and his family were supported by his father in law for ten years. Within that period Raphael was expected to become an outstanding rabbi or judge on a rabbinical court or similar prominent position. Raphael's peers were brilliant too, so there was no way to feel outstanding. Moreover, his entire education warned against pride and inculcated modesty. Raphael himself had acknowledged that his brilliance as a scholar derived from his genes, the care and education he had received from his parents and Providence: he only had to work hard in order not to fail expectations. Nonetheless, Raphael was just as human as anyone else; he probably unloaded at home some of the great pressure he faced in the yeshiva. I saw how Rivka softly started to cry, but this time it seemed to me the cry of relief, as if her isolation was broken, as if someone, including Raphael finally, finally understood her feelings.

When Dr. Jacobs joined, I gave him a brief account of the conversation in front of the young couple. I briefly stated some of the main facts, which we already had discussed in my room. Repeating a patient's life story in his presence is a sign that one has listened carefully. But recounting some of the meaningful insights that surfaced during the patient-doctor interview has a real therapeutic benefit. Raphael's eyes were glued on me during this brief review, while Rivka's shifted between her husband and the doctors standing at the foot of her bed. "In conclusion, Dr. Jacobs it seems to me that we are dealing with two outstanding persons, the woman not less than her husband. Both are superb followers of God's commands and each tries to live up to the highest moral expectations, but occasionally they fail. Fortunately, they know that each downturn is destined to be followed by an upturn. And fortunately they know the deeper significance of trials, to which every human being is subjected. It seems to me that each of this marvelous couple needs a wise companion of their own gender to provide guidance regarding various practical aspects of marriage. Finally, Dr. Jacobs, I believe this couple actually needed the present predicament to help them grow in theory *and* practice in order to prepare them for their future responsibilities".

After appropriate arrangements had been made the Shuchats were discharged from hospital. I felt some satisfaction that a psychiatric admission had been averted and that this couple was probably guided onto an appropriate path of development. The most important work had to be done by the couple themselves and the reward of their efforts would be theirs and theirs only. In the busy hospital one patient follows the other and my attention was soon drawn to other patients. The Shuchats' case joined that of others: as a marked sticker in my book.

About one year later I found a voice mail message from Raphael. When I called, he reassured me straightaway. Thank God Rivka was alright and actually thriving, they had recently started the obstetric process of having a new pregnancy and the children were healthy and well. Both had received guidance for several months from a rabbi and his wife, who specialized in marriage counsel. However, something new had developed in their lives, on the borderline between medicine and spirituality and Raphael wondered whether he could consult with me. Could anyone expect that I would refuse such a request?

Raphael looked unchanged, his eyes sparkling with brilliance, his face and body language expressing modesty and refined behavior. He belonged clearly to the best of the best that yeshiva culture had produced over the last two or three millennia. Interestingly, Raphael had decided he wished to consult with a doctor rather than with his rabbi, the choice by default of most yeshiva students. Although he had initiated this meeting, he evidently needed to conjure up the courage to start. Possibly I looked different than the idealized mental picture in his memory and mind, formed during those stressful days of one year ago. He started in a soft voice, carefully framing each sentence. "You know, God bless much has changed since last year. We have both benefited from the close counsel we received after Rivka's discharge from hospital. I have read and enjoyed the book that you recommended and it has opened my eyes on more than one issue. I think we better understand the various tasks we have to fulfill to make the marriage and the home function appropriately". He paused for a second or two and I sensed he was about to divulge his punch line, the reason for his visit. "Just when you expect you deserve a present for your efforts, you get the opposite. I have received a measure for a measure". He looked down, possibly embarrassed, possibly hoping I would read his veiled language.

Raphael had referred to a basic concept in the Torah, i.e. that man reaps according to what one sows. The Torah is replete with stories that demonstrate how punishment is meted out exactly according to the parameters of the initial offense. One year ago, Raphael had confessed of two "sins": being exceedingly jealous of his wife and having coerced his wife to marital relations one day before she was due to immerse in the ritual bath. During the subsequent three-way conversation at Rivka's bedside he had more or less realized that his frequent criticism had been a major source of depression for his wife. So which punishment could he have received that served as measure against measure? Had his wife become jealous of him, and how did that possibly manifest? Perhaps she had become critical of her husband: not unlikely, the received guidance could have empowered her to make demands of her husband that were perhaps quite reasonable, but unexpected by her husband. After all, as a child prodigy and ever since he had been pampered and all technical aspects of life were taking care of by others in order to facilitate and support his studies. Although these events might have occurred, they were probably not the reason for his request to come and see me. After all, he had mentioned a problem on the borderline between medicine and spirituality. A sexual issue seemed more probable, which also would explain his veiled language. A sexuality transmitted disease seemed highly unlikely, given this man's high moral quality, but everything is possible. A problem with sexual performance seemed more likely.

Indirect language should be met similarly. "Raphael, are you possibly referring to some difficulty with carrying out your marital obligations?" The Ketubah or marriage contract, which every Jewish male signs at his wedding, specifies the husband's obligations towards his wife: to provide for her and the family's needs, to honor her, to work for her and also to have marital relations. Raphael acknowledged: "One year ago I made an unreasonable and un-Halachic demand of my wife: in the last two months I have twice been unable to do my duty. And both times were after Rivka went to immerse in the ritual bath". After a pause he added: "She was actually very wise and understanding. God bless and at other times things have worked as usual. Nonetheless, I fail to fulfill the command of relations after my wife's ritual immersion. And I worry that at my young age I cope with such a problem – although I recognize the measure for measure punishment".

Reassuring Raphael was the easy part. A medical problem could easily be ruled out. I had heard about this phenomenon: some men, who are otherwise saintly followers of the Halachah simply cannot stand the command to have marital relations on that one particular day in the monthly calendar. They evidently feel that relations should take place upon their initiative and there is a special thrill in encountering the wife's reluctance and then appeasing her into agreement. "However Raphael, as both of us know, there is always a deeper layer behind that what meets our eye. One such layer is a certain inability or unwillingness to bend our will before the commands of the law. You know with your head - perhaps not yet with your heart, but you will grow into that - that the laws of family purity all serve the physical and spiritual health of the couple. Abstinence of all physical contact during about twelve days each month is a challenge, especially for men, but it helps conquer one's base instincts and induces psychological and spiritual growth. However, I suspect we are dealing with an additional and very personal layer". He looked questioningly and I continued but only after he confirmed that he wished me to.

The Torah tells the fast-paced story of Jacob and his flight to his uncle Laban after Jacob's brother Esaph vows to murder him. He arrives penniless with Laban, who has two daughters. The eldest is Leah, who has "soft eyes", while her younger sister Rachel is described as being beautiful. Jacob loves Rachel and undertakes to work for his uncle for seven years instead of paying a dowry. When the time has come, Laban throws a party and subsequently in the dark brings his veiled daughter Lea to Jacob. Unwittingly, Jacob consummates the marriage and only the next day he recognizes the deceit. When he files his strong protest with Laban the latter provides a pathetic excuse: it is not customary in their location to have the younger daughter marry before the older one. However, Laban convinces Jacob to sit out that week and he will receive his beloved Rachel in marriage too, albeit at the price of having to work for him for another seven years. These are the plain facts of the story. Anyone unfamiliar with this story would have guessed that Jacob's marriage of love with Rachel would be happy and productive, whereas the forced marriage with Lea would be sterile. The reality was quite the opposite. The Torah states that Lea was hated, while Rachel's womb was closed. Nonetheless, Lea gave birth to six sons and one daughter, while Rachel remained childless for fourteen years until Joseph was born and when his brother Benjamin was born six years later she died in childbirth.

There is a Talmudic tractate wondering about God's actions after he has created the world. Has God created the world, rested on the seventh day and then retired from the world He created? According to the Jewish understanding God remains very much involved in all details of the world. In particular, He arranges the matches between men and women, which is a notoriously difficult affair. Now when Jacob, or for that matter every other man, choses the woman of his heart, is that his own choice or the result of God's matchmaking? The following Hassidic interpretation of Jacob's saga with his wives is enlightening. While Jacob married two wives, the loved Rachel and the unloved Lea, most men nowadays marry one woman at the time. They start out by marrying the woman they love, their Rachel, but invariably and usually within several years they recognize Lea aspects in their wife that they profoundly dislike. Friction and tensions start and, handled un-expertly may lead to estrangement or divorce. Handed with wisdom, patience, humility and perseverance, the short-lived fall-in-love phase makes way for a much deeper and durable love for the remainder of one's life. It seems that man himself chooses the lovely Rachel component, while God attaches the unseen and hated Lea component as part of the deal. Looking at the biblical story, one wonders how Jacob's union with Lea after such an abysmal start could have become so extraordinary fertile. The only possible answer to this question is that both partners invested a great deal in time, attention and conversation to make their marriage work. Finally, the Rachel component of every marriage is doomed to be sterile – although it serves as essential bridge to the second, more important and longer-lasting Lea phase of the relationship.

"It seems to me, Raphael that you are in the transitory phase. You have been married for several years and your angelic Rachel has started manifesting some Lea components. You confirmed that your wife has made extensive use of the expert guidance from a Rabbi's wife and continues to do so – while after several meetings you have discontinued seeking this Rabbi's counsel. Your wife is probably learning how to set limits to her husband's behavior and wishes, which is exactly what a righteous woman is supposed to do. You know, Raphael, adult men are not unlike young boys, expecting that our wishes and whims are met. While boys love games, adult men crave material goods including money, pleasure and social recognition and honor. It is not unheard of that famous men, both in secular and religious capacities, have huge social standing but at home there is much marital discord. These men spend too little time and attention on their families and too much on the road in a subconscious quest for honor or power or they may be addicted to feeling essential to others. You may experience your wife's growing but legitimate demands for your time and support of your family's requirements as restricting your development. Possibly you feel anger or frustration; not unlikely these feelings are suppressed and are not readily accessible to you. However, our bodies are the instrument on which our soul plays its music and expresses itself. The symptom that brought you to see me is a classic example of a subconscious feeling of frustration expressing itself in physical form".

Raphael had been listening with concentration and attention. Here and there he interrupted me, in particular to quote verbatim the biblical texts I mentioned. He had scribbled several catch words in order not to interrupt me and then asked two questions. First, how do you know if your wife's requests are legitimate or if she is becoming too demanding? Second, how do you make that transition between the two phases of your marriage? I congratulated him for asking excellent questions, but refrained from entering into a detailed discussion. These issues should be extensively discussed with a therapist or professional counselor. Rather than a theoretical one-time talk, Raphael should raise real-life examples and his counselor could provide him with insight and practical advice. The common ground between his two questions was the newly gained insight regarding the necessity to work on his marriage.

"Raphael, there are two final comments I would like to make before you leave. First, it is not only your marriage which has to make the transition between a superficial initial phase to a mature lasting form. It is also you yourself who has to transform from an intellectual powerhouse into a mature, experienced and wise man. You should accordingly view the crisis period last year, the current difficulties at home and the symptom that brought you to see me as unique means for transformation. Ultimately, the rectified man strives to resemble God, changing from a young man out to *obtain* satisfaction for his wishes into a benevolent wise person, who seeks to *give*: material, emotional and spiritual gifts in first instance to his wife and children and then to ever-wider social circles". Raphael indicated that he was familiar with this idea, although he now felt and experienced how the actual process took place. And the second comment?

"Raphael, like every human being you have been presented with certain problems and symptoms. Last year you discovered that at the root of two problems, which you experienced as sins and were much ashamed of, were the horror of nothingness and fear of death. I congratulated you for your intellectual and emotional work, without which you would not have been able to get at these little devils in the basement of your soul and also for your honesty to share with me, a doctor. Although I recommended that you go and start working on these issues, you choose to ignore them like most people do in such circumstances. Perhaps the best way is to consider these frightening themes in our lives as gifts from Heaven, because they provide a window to the innermost layers of our soul. Like I mentioned at your wife's bedside one year ago, you could and perhaps should embrace these difficulties in the knowledge that they have been presented to you as a means to make you grow in experience and wisdom – and help you prepare for your future responsibilities in life. Please avail yourself of one of the possible counselors I pointed out to you and get serious at working on these personal issues. I don't doubt that your superb theoretical knowledge of the Torah and its precepts will serve as ladder to emotional and spiritual growth – while simultaneously providing you with a greater depth of understanding of the Torah than previously possible".

Epilogue

Occasionally people meet who have not seen each other for a long time. During that initial fraction of a moment they search each other's face, looking for signs of aging. In case they don't find such, and sometimes also if they do, they may make their friend a compliment by saying that he or she has not changed at all. This, of course, implies that no apparent change is commendable and perhaps that the friend may achieve older age, while remaining young at heart. However, man alone among all creatures knows his eventual demise. His response to that knowledge alternates from denial, to anxiety, to acceptance with additional in-between stages. Western society celebrates youth and outward beauty. But what about the splendor of a grey-bearded, wise old man? Or the soft and kind understanding eyes in the wrinkled face of a grandmother? Life *is* change; definitions of life all refer to metabolism, or a turnover of substances, which lies at the heart of all life forms. The western approach to life is outward oriented: doing and acting is the ostentatious means and purpose of everything, and success is defined by the number and kind of creations produced. We all know that there is an inner aspect of life, with pains, love, anxieties, unfulfilled wishes, dreams and nightmares. However, these feelings do not receive outward attention. Although they are present all the time, keep buzzing during the day and especially at night, they are often considered a distraction, which keep us from fully expressing our abilities. They are considered, more or less a nuisance.

There is, however, a different attitude to life. In this totally different approach, man's inner being occupies center place. In this view, the world serves as stage to help educate the soul. Every single action in this exterior theater is accompanied by events within the soul of the protagonists, leading to inner progress. Moreover, every single action in the world is also the *result* of inner forces. In this view, the soul is born in order to complete itself, to grow and educate itself and this process can only be accomplished by living in a down-to-earth world. People subscribing to the outward oriented view of life as well as those with the inward looking approach live and act in the real world. However, the former consider that at its purpose, while the latter as a means: a means to inner growth and development. In the latter view, everything that happens, even unpleasant things, serve a positive purpose, to help the involved person grow and develop. Change is of necessity the means to achieve growth and lack of change is a sign of stagnation. Nonetheless, most people hate and resist change. Perhaps, maybe often, they are not too happy with their life the way it is, but they have become accustomed to it and prefer the inadequacies of their life rather than have any changes with their inherent uncertainty regarding outcome. Judaism calls this mindset one of bondage and banishment, while man is destined to freedom and the path to it involves active transformation as well as uncertainty. Only a true belief that this is one's destiny will empower a person to overcome his inherent aversion to change and stick to his unique, untraveled road.

It is the doctor's mandate to help cure the patient and relieve suffering. However, heal only the physical component? Is that all there is? The eminent psychologist Carl G. Jung hypothesized that the Western world maintained a complot against man's inner life. If there is heart disease, or diabetes, or an infection, does that mean that the problem concerns the relevant body systems only? Even the most level headed physician acknowledges that a physical disease *causes* changes in an individual's life such as the need to take medication, impose physical limitations and looking differently at life. Physicians act as if those inner, emotional components are none of their business, rather something personal. Even more, the idea that perhaps an illness *originated* from some deeper, emotional or spiritual source sounds at first hand outrageous. However, all doctors acknowledge that smoking, alcohol, drugs, overeating and lack of physical exercise cause various diseases. Even if certain genes predispose to certain diseases, behavioral and environmental factors do influence the extent to which certain genes are expressed. The onset of a disease on the one hand is the culmination of an inner process that finally manifests in physical symptoms. On the other hand, it may lead to awareness regarding the source of the illness and a behavioral change may lead to cure or prevent additional physical ailments. Physicians should **dare** to refer to the inner reflection - or causes - of physical ailments and encourage their patients to accost and transform these inner issues. Acknowledgement of the need for change in the patient of necessity leads to change and growth in the doctor himself. A doctor who has worked on his own issues and problems is much more effective for his patients.

It is notoriously difficult to change as all acknowledge who have battled with smoking, drinking, drugs, overeating, womanizing, etc or have taken care of patients who faced these problems. However, to paraphrase a common saying: man's tendency to materialism makes transformation necessary, while his inclination to spirituality makes it possible.

The patient recognizes that he is more than a body. His body is a vehicle for his individuality and specialness. A non- or inappropriately functioning body does not allow a full expression of a person's individuality. Therefore, any disease mandates intervention that should lead to transformation. Perhaps it is not a physician's task to fully explore all inner aspects of a physical ailment. However, a total denial of this component alienates the patient. It is the golden hour of opportunity to direct a patient. At the moment of his greatest pain and concern he is most open to suggestions to have a new, fresh look at himself and within himself. This is what a doctor needs learn to do, and needs to do. Put the patient on a new path, show him the light, to be followed by specialist assistance of various kinds, or just by himself and his spouse.

Real health is not only an absence of illness. It is an appropriate development and expression of the true self, a complete alignment of the soul, body and society, and the recognition of God within himself and everywhere.

Alphabetical list of Hebrew words and their explanation:

Ashkenazim: Jews of European descent.

Bar Mitswah: After his thirteenth birthday a Jewish boy is presumed to be acknowledgeable enough to be responsible for his deeds and follow the Torah's commands or precepts. This birthday is especially celebrated.

Chafetz Chaim: Literally "Lover of Life," although "Someone who appreciates life" more appropriately conveys the author's intend. The author of the book is Rabbi Israel Meir of Radin, nicknamed after his book Chafetz Chaim.

Halachah: Code of Jewish Law and conduct.

Haredy: ultra-orthodox section of modern Jewry.

Ketuba: marriage contract, which the Jewish husband signs at his marriage with witnesses as counter signers.

Làmah: Hebrew for "why".

Lemàh: Hebrew for "for what purpose".

Midrash: Large body of stories and legends, dating back to the time of Abraham up to the time of the writing of the Talmud in the fifth century CE.

Mitswah: The 613 precepts or commands as written in the Torah.

Rebbe: The central religious and moral authority in Hassidic communities, whom is consulted regarding all important decisions in life.

Sephardim: Jews originating from Spain, Portugal, North African or Arab or Asian countries.

Shiva: the seven days of obligatory mourning at home when a close family member has passed away.

Tikun: literally mean repair or amendment. This central Jewish concept indicates that people can and should amend their deficiencies throughout their lives.

Torah: The Pentateuch or five books of Moses.

Yeshiva: Religious seminary.

Biography and references

Introduction:
1. Hesse H. Narcissus and Goldmund. Picador, US, 1968.
2. Cronin AJ. The Citadel. A Back Bay book, USA.
3. Munthe A. The story of San Michele. Flamingo, HarperCollins, London UK, 1995.
4. Camus A. The plague. Penguin books, UK, 1971.
5. Kleinman A. The illness narratives. Suffering, healing and the human condition. Perseus, Basic Books, USA 1988.
6. Leader D, Corfield D. Why do people get ill? Penguin books, UK, 2008.
7. Halevy J. Complementary and alternative medicine. All the facts. (Hebrew) Kinneret, Zmora-Bitan, Dvir – Publishing House, Ltd.2005.
8. Stettbacher JK. Making sense of suffering. The healing confrontation with your own past. Penguin books, USA 1991.
9. Matalon A, Rabin S. Behind the consultation. Reflective stories from clinical practice. Radcliffe publishing, UK 2007.
10. Maoz B, Rabin S, Katz H, Matalon A. The patient and the doctor and their interactions. An introduction to relational medicine. (Hebrew). The Tel Aviv University 2004.
11. Rabin S, Maoz B, Shorer Y, Matalon A. Rekindling the spirit; creativity, passion and the prevention of burnout in the medical profession. (Hebrew) Tel Aviv University, 2010.
12. Sacks O. The man who mistook his wife for a hat. Picador, London UK, 1985.
13. Hospital Medicine (Part 1): what is wrong with acute hospital care? Eur J Intern Med. 2009;20:462-4.
14. Heyman SN, Ben Yehuda A, Brezis M. Additional remedies for the failing departments of internal medicine. Harefuah. 2010;149:756-7, 813. Hebrew.
15. Julian K, Riegels NS, Baron RB. Perspective: Creating the next generation of general internists: a call for medical education reform. Acad Med. 2011;86:1443-7.
16. Warner JH. The humanizing power of medical history: responses to biomedicine in the 20th century United States. Med Humanit. 2011;37:91-6.
17. Gaufberg EH, Batalden M, Sands R, Bell SK. The hidden curriculum: what can we learn from third-year medical student narrative reflections? Acad Med. 2010;85:1709-16.
18. Sturgeon D. 'Have a nice day': consumerism, compassion and health care. Br J Nurs. 2010;19:1047-51.
19. Ghadirian AM. Is spirituality relevant to the practice of medicine? Med Law. 2008; 27:229-39.
20. Keall RM, Butow PN, Steinhauser KE, Clayton JM. Discussing life story, forgiveness, heritage, and legacy with patients with life-limiting illnesses. Int J Palliat Nurs. 2011;17:454-60.
21. College of physicians and surgeons, Columbia University. Narrative medicine workshops.
22. Scott JG, Scott RG, Miller WL, Stange KC, Crabtree BF. Healing relationships and the existential philosophy of Martin Buber. Ethic Humanities Med 2009; 4: 11.
23. Egnew TR. The meaning of healing: transcending suffering. Ann Fam Med 2005; 3: 255-262.
24. Egnew TR. Suffering, meaning and healing: challenges of contemporary medicine. Ann Fam Med 2009; 7: 170-175.

Chapter 1. Symptoms as symbols: The woman with the broken arm.
1. Jung CG. Man and his symbols. Arkana, Penguin Group, 1990.
2. Bible: Exodus.
3. Szyk A. Roth C, editor. The (Passover) Haggadah. Massadah & Alumoth, Jerusalem, Israel 1957.

4. Zalman Rabbi Schneur. Likutei Amarim -Tanya. Bi-lingual edition. "Kehot" Publication Society. Brooklyn NY, 1993.
5. Rabbi Nahman. Likutei Moharan (Hebrew).
6. Blomberg BB, Alvarez JP, Diaz A, et al. Psychosocial adaptation and cellular immunity in breast cancer patients in the weeks after surgery: An exploratory study. J Psychosom Res. 2009;67:369-76.
7. Hernandez-Reif M, Ironson G, Field T, et al. Breast cancer patients have improved immune and neuroendocrine functions following massage therapy. J Psychosom Res. 2004;57:45-52.
8. Castilla-Cortázar I, Castilla A, Gurpegui M. Opioid peptides and immunodysfunction in patients with major depression and anxiety disorders. J Physiol Biochem. 1998;54:203-15.
9. Gennaro S, Fehder WP, Cnaan A, et al. Immune responses in mothers of term and preterm very-low-birth-weight infants. Clin Diagn Lab Immunol. 1997;4:565-71.
10. Extein I, Tallman J, Smith CC, Goodwin FK. Changes in lymphocyte beta-adrenergic receptors in depression and mania. Psychiatry Res. 1979;1:191-7.
11. Kark JD, Goldman S, Epstein L. Iraqi missile attacks on Israel. The association of mortality with a life-threatening stressor. JAMA. 1995;273:1208-10.
12. Stroebe M, Schut H, Stroebe W. Health outcomes of bereavement. Lancet. 2007; 370: 1960-73.

Chapter 2. Making sense of suffering: The baby with end stage renal disease.

1. Weiss BL: Many lives, many masters. A fireside book. Simon & Schuster, NY 1988.
2. Frankl VE. Man's search for meaning.Washington Square Press, NY 1984.
3. Haich E. Initiation. Aurora Press, Santa Fe, NM, USA 2000.
4. Vogt BA, Avner ED. Renal failure. In: Kliegman RM, Behrman RE, Jenson HB, Stanton BF, eds. Nelson Textbook of Pediatrics. 18th ed. Saunders Elsevier 2007; 2206-2214.
5. Illness and identity. Seifter JL. Am J Kidney Dis. 2011;58:A22-4.
6. Hendrickson KC. Morbidity, mortality, and parental grief: a review of the literature on the relationship between the death of a child and the subsequent health of parents. Palliat Support Care. 2009;7:109-19.
7. Sychev D, Maya ID, Allon M. Clinical outcomes of dialysis catheter-related candidemia in hemodialysis patients. Clin J Am Soc Nephrol. 2009;4:1102-5.
8. Blyth CC, Chen SC, Slavin MA, et al. Not just little adults: candidemia epidemiology, molecular characterization, and antifungal susceptibility in neonatal and pediatric patients. Australian Candidemia Study. Pediatrics. 2009;123:1360-8.
9. Beil S, Drube J, Gluer S, Lehner F, Ehrich JH, Pape L. End-stage renal disease due to ARPKD in the first months of life: transplantation or dialysis?--two case reports. Pediatr Transplant. 2010;14:E75-8.
10. Carey WA, Talley LI, Sehring SA, Jaskula JM, Mathias RS. Outcomes of dialysis initiated during the neonatal period for treatment of end-stage renal disease: a North American Pediatric Renal Trials and Collaborative Studies special analysis. Pediatrics. 2007;119:e468-73.
11. Dolbec K, Mick NW. Congenital heart disease. Emerg Med Clin North Am. 2011;29:811-27, vii. Review.
12. Loriedo C, Torti C. Systemic hypnosis with depressed individuals and their families. Int J Clin Exp Hypn. 2010;58:222-46.
13. Tong A, Lowe A, Sainsbury P, Craig JC. Experiences of parents who have children with chronic kidney disease: a systematic review of qualitative studies. Pediatrics. 2008;121:349-60.

Chapter 3: Futile medicine? The elderly, dement patient on the respirator.
1. Mandell LA, Wunderink R. Pneumonia. In: Longo DL, Fauci AS, Kaspar DL, Hauser SL, Jameson JL, Loscalzo J, eds. Harrison's Principles and Practice of Internal Medicine. 18st edition. McGraw Hill NY 2012; 2130-2141.
2. Musher D. Streptococcus pneumoniae. In: Mandell GL, Bennett JE, Dolin R, eds. Mandell, Douglas and Bennett's Principles and Practice of Infectious Diseases. 7th edition. Churchill Livingstone Elsevier, Philadelphia 2010: 2623-42.
3. Spence D. Advance directives. BMJ. 2011 Nov 2
4. Esayag Y, Nikitin I, Bar-Ziv J, et al. Diagnostic value of chest radiographs in bedridden patients suspected of having pneumonia. Am J Med 2010; 123: 88.e1-88.e6
5. Pugh R, Grant C, Cooke RP, Dempsey G. Short-course versus prolonged-course antibiotic therapy for hospital-acquired pneumonia in critically ill adults. Cochrane Database Syst Rev. 2011 5:CD007577.
6. Zilberberg V, Shorr AF. Ventilator-associated pneumonia as a model for approaching cost-effectiveness and infection prevention in the ICU. Curr Opin Infect Dis. 2011;24:385-9.
7. Burns JP, Truog RD. Futility: a concept in evolution. Chest 2007;132:1987-93..
8. Albar MA. Saudi J. Seeking remedy, abstaining from therapy and resuscitation: an Islamic perspective. Kidney Dis Transpl. 2007;18:629-37.
9. Luce JM. A history of resolving conflicts over end-of-life care in intensive care units in the United States. Crit Care Med. 2010;38:1623-9.

Chapter 4: A hole in his heart
1. Jung CG. Synchronicity. An Acausal connection principle.
2. Jung CG. Memories, dreams and reflections.
3. Fowler VG, Scheld WM, Bayer AS. Endocarditis and intravascular infections. In: Mandell GL, Bennett JE, Dolin R, eds. Mandell, Douglas and Bennett's Principles and Practice of Infectious Diseases. 7th edition. Churchill Livingstone Elsevier, Philadelphia 2010: 1067-1112.
4. Solomon M, Raveh D, Yinnon M. Assessment of physicians' knowledge of guidelines for the prevention of infective endocarditis. J Hosp Infect 2000;45:311-317.
5. Feffer P, Raveh D, Schlesinger Y, Rudensky B, Yinnon AM. Determination of number of blood cultures required for diagnosis of infective endocarditis: Review of 108 consecutive patients from a 10-year period (1990-1999). Eur J Clin Microbiol Infect Dis 2002; 21: 432-7.
6. Shapiro N, Merin O, Rosenmann E, Dzigivker I, Bitran D, Yinnon AM, Silberman S. Prevalence and epidemiology of unsuspected endocarditis detected after elective valve replacement. Ann Thorac Surg 2004; 78: 1623-9.
7. Wiener-Well Y, Schlesinger Y, Raveh D, Fink D, Yinnon AM. Q fever endocarditis: not always expected. Clin Microbiol Infect 2010; 16: 359-362
8. Meerkin D, Yinnon AM, Munter RG, Shemesh O, Abraham AS. Mycotic aneurysm of the aortic arch due to Salmonella group D. Case report and review of the literature. Clin Infect Dis 1995; 21: 523-8.
9. Raveh D, Schlesinger Y, Rudensky B, Yinnon AM. Prosthetic valve endocarditis due to Listeria monocytogenes. Inf Dis Clin Pract 1998; 7: 351-353.
10. Benenson S, Raveh D, Schlesinger Y, et al. The risk of vascular infection in adult patients with non-typhi Salmonella endocarditis. Am J Med 2001; 110:60-3.
11. Lo Rito M, Leon-Wyss J, Veras O, Vides I, Najera C, Castañeda AR. Antibiotic sandwich patch for ventricular septal defect complicated by endocarditis.Ann Thorac Surg. 2011;92:366-8.
12. Penny DJ, Vick GW 3rd. Ventricular septal defect. Lancet. 2011;377:1103-12.

13. Chessa M, Butera G, Negura D, et al. Transcatheter closure of congenital ventricular septal defects in adult: mid-term results and complications. Int J Cardiol 2009;133:70-3.

Chapter 5: More futile medicine? Reading between the lines.
1. Kushner HS. When bad things happen to good people. Anchor Books. NY 1981.
2. Genesis 4: 3-8: Cain and Abel.
3. Exodus 30:34-36: Preparation of incense.
4. Biblical Book Esther.
5. Yalom ID: Momma and the meaning of life. Tales of psychotherapy. Basic Books, 1999.
6. Jotkowitz A. Feeding patients with advanced dementia: a Jewish ethical perspective. J Clin Ethics. 2004;15:346-9.
7. Lee KF. Postoperative futile care: stopping the train when the family says "keep going". Thorac Surg Clin. 2005;15:481-91.
8. Wijdicks EF, Rabinstein AA. Absolutely no hope? Some ambiguity of futility of care in devastating acute stroke. Crit Care Med. 2004;32:2332-42.
9. Shapiro DS, Friedmann R. To feed or not to feed the terminal demented patient--is there any question? Isr Med Assoc J. 2006;8:507-8.
10. Raveh D, Gratch L, Yinnon AM, Sonnenblick M. Demographic and clinical characteristics of patients admitted to medical departments. J Eval Clin Pract. 2005;11:33-44.
11. Sonnenblick M, Gratch L, Raveh D, Steinberg A, Yinnon AM. Epidemiology of decision on life-sustaining treatment in the general internal medicine division. Harefuah. 2003;142:650-3, 720. Hebrew.
12. Thinnes A, Padilla R. Effect of educational and supportive strategies on the ability of caregivers of people with dementia to maintain participation in that role. Am J Occup Ther. 2011;65:541-9.
13. Letts L, Edwards M, Berenyi J, et al. Using occupations to improve quality of life, health and wellness, and client and caregiver satisfaction for people with Alzheimer's disease and related dementias. Am J Occup Ther. 201;65:497-504.
14. Joseph R. Hospital policy on medical futility - does it help in conflict resolution and ensuring good end-of-life care? Ann Acad Med Singapore. 2011;40:19-7.
15. van Vliet D, de Vugt ME, Bakker C, Koopmans RT, Verhey FR. Impact of early onset dementia on caregivers: a review. Int J Geriatr Psychiatry. 2010;25:1091-100.
16. Etters L, Goodall D, Harrison BE. Caregiver burden among dementia patient caregivers: a review of the literature. J Am Acad Nurse Pract. 2008;20:423-8.

Chapter 6: Perforated bowel: The unexpected benefit of a second opinion
1. Gawande A. Complications: A surgeon's notes on an imperfect science. Picadot, 2002.
2. Groopman. How doctors think. A Mariner Book. Houghton Mifflin Company. Boston, 2008.
3. Gearhart SL. Diverticular disease and common anorectal disorders. In Fauci AS, Braunwald E, Kaspar DL, Hauser SL, Longo DL, Jameson JL, Loscalzo J, eds. Harrison's Principles and practice of internal medicine, 17th edition. McGrawHill Medical, NY, 2008:1903-9.
4. Goldman RE, Sullivan A, Back AL, et al. Patients' reflections on communication in the second-opinion hematology-oncology consultation. Patient Educ Couns 2009; 76: 44–50.
5. Lantos J, Matlock AM, Wendler D. Clinician integrity and limits to patient autonomy. JAMA. 2011;305:495-9.
6. Lahey T, Shah R, Gittzus J, Schwartzman J, Kirkland K. Infectious diseases consultation lowers mortality from Staphylococcus aureus bacteremia. Medicine (Baltimore). 2009;88:263-7.

7. Yinnon AM. Whither infectious diseases consultations? Analysis of 14,005 consultations from a five year period in a general hospital. Clin Infect Dis 2001; 33: 1661-7.
8. Vermeulen J, van der Harst E, Lange JF. Pathophysiology and prevention of diverticulitis and perforation. Neth J Med. 2010;68:303-9.
9. Jaffer U, Moin T. Perforated sigmoid diverticular disease: a management protocol. JSLS. 2008;12:188-93.
10. Flasar MH, Goldberg E. Acute abdominal pain. Med Clin North Am. 2006;90:481-503.
11. White SI, Frenkiel B, Martin PJ. A ten-year audit of perforated sigmoid diverticulitis: highlighting the outcomes of laparoscopic lavage. Dis Colon Rectum. 2010;53:1537-41.
12. Faith K, Chidwick P. Role of clinical ethicists in making decisions about levels of care in the intensive care unit. Crit Care Nurse. 2009;29:77-84.

Chapter 7. CMV in pregnancy: counseling with wisdom in the face of uncertainty

1. Genesis 22: 1. Abraham's tribulations.
2. Crumpacker CS II, Zhang JL. Cytomegalovirus. In: Mandell GL, Bennett JE, Dolin R, eds. Mandell, Douglas and Bennett's Principles and Practice of Infectious Diseases. 7th edition. Churchill Livingstone Elsevier, Philadelphia 2010: 1971-87.
3. Lazzarotto T, Guerra B, Gabrielli L, Lanari M, Landini MP. Update on the prevention, diagnosis and management of cytomegalovirus during pregnancy. Clin Microbiol Infect 2011; 17: 1285-1293.
4. Johannsen EC, Kaye KM. Epstein-Barr virus (Infectious mononucleosis, Epstein-Barr Virus-associated malignant diseases, and other diseases). In: Mandell GL, Bennett JE, Dolin R, eds. Mandell, Douglas and Bennett's Principles and Practice of Infectious Diseases. 7th edition. Churchill Livingstone Elsevier, Philadelphia 2010: 1989-2010.
5. Wiener-Well Y, Yinnon AM, Singer P, Hersch M. Reactivation of cytomegalovirus in critically sick patients. Isr Med Assoc J 2006; 8: 583-4.
6. Yinnon AM. The case for routine screening of Cytomegalovirus before pregnancy: counseling with wisdom in the face of uncertainty (Invited Editorial). IMAJ 207; 9: 391.
7. Early-life environment influencing susceptibility to cytomegalovirus infection: evidence from the Leiden Longevity Study and the Longitudinal Study of Aging Danish Twins. Mortensen LH, Maier AB, Slagbom PE, et al. Epidemiol Infect. 2011 Jul 25:1-7.
8. Gindes L, Teperberg-Oikawa M, Sherman D, Pardo J, Rahav G. Congenital cytomegalovirus infection following primary maternal infection in the third trimester. BJOG. 2008;115:830-5.
9. Rahav G, Gabbay R, Ornoy A, Shechtman S, Arnon J, Diav-Citrin O. Primary versus nonprimary cytomegalovirus infection during pregnancy, Israel. Emerg Infect Dis. 2007;13:1791-3.
10. Schlesinger Y. Routine screening for CMV in pregnancy: opening the Pandora box? Isr Med Assoc J. 2007;9:395-7.
11. Schlesinger Y, Reich D, Eidelman AI, Schimmel MS, Hassanin J, Miron D. Congenital cytomegalovirus infection in Israel: screening in different subpopulations. Isr Med Assoc J. 2005;7:237-40.
12. Schlesinger Y, Halle D, Eidelman AI, et al. Urine polymerase chain reaction as a screening tool for the detection of congenital cytomegalovirus infection. Arch Dis Child Fetal Neonatal Ed. 2003;88:F371-4.
13. Schimmel MS, Fisher D, Schlesinger Y. J Perinatol. Congenital cytomegalovirus infection (CMV). 2001;21:209-10.

Chapter 8: Sexually transmitted infection: fertile ground for personal development
1. Yalom ID. The Schopenhauer cure. Harper Collins Publishers, 2005.
2. Ginsburgh, Rabbi Y. Body, mind and soul. Kabbalah on human physiology, disease and healing. Gal Einai Institute, Inc. 2003.
3. Glazerson M. Torah, light and healing. Mystical insight into healing based on the Hebrew language. Jason Aronson, Inc, 1996.
4. Sherman IW. Twelve diseases that changed our world. ASM press, Washington DC, 2007.
5. Cartwright FE, Biddiss MD. Disease and history. Barnes & Noble, NY 1972.
6. Genesis: 38: 1-30. Tamar and Jehuda.
7. Amnon and Tamar. 2 Samuel 13.
8. Bible. Hosea Chapter 1-3. Hosea's tragedy.
9. Frankel E: Sacred therapy. Shambhala Publications, Inc 2003.
10. Sacks O. Awakenings. Picador, UK 1991.
11. Marrazzo JM, Handsfield HH, Sparkling PF. Neisseria gonorrhoeae. In: Mandell GL, Bennett JE, Dolin R, eds. Mandell, Douglas and Bennett's Principles and Practice of Infectious Diseases. 7th edition. Churchill Livingstone Elsevier, Philadelphia 2010: 2753-70.
12. Tramont EC. Treponema pallidum (Syphilis). In: Mandell GL, Bennett JE, Dolin R, eds. Mandell, Douglas and Bennett's Principles and Practice of Infectious Diseases. 7th edition. Churchill Livingstone Elsevier, Philadelphia 2010: 3035-53.
13. Acquired immunodeficiency syndrome. In: Mandell GL, Bennett JE, Dolin R, eds. Mandell, Douglas and Bennett's Principles and Practice of Infectious Diseases. 7th edition. Churchill Livingstone Elsevier, Philadelphia 2010: 1619-1895.
14. Yinnon AM, Coury-Doniger P, Polito R, Reichman RC. Serologic response to treatment of syphilis in patients with HIV- infection. Arch Intern Med 156: 321-325, 1996.
15. Yinnon AM, Klutstein MW, Balkin J. Gonococcal endocarditis: A rare disease. Isr J Med Sci 1988; 24: 429-430.
16. Mor Z, Goor Y, de Musquita SB, Shohat T. The Levinsky walk-in clinic in Tel Aviv: holistic services to control sexually transmitted diseases in the community. Harefuah. 2010;149:503-7, 551. Hebrew.
17. Carey MP, Senn TE, Vanable PA, Coury-Doniger P, Urban MA. Brief and intensive behavioral interventions to promote sexual risk reduction among STD clinic patients: results from a randomized controlled trial. AIDS Behav. 2010;14:504-17.
18. Manavi K. The features of patients attending walk-in compared with booked clinics for sexually transmitted infections. Int J STD AIDS. 2007;18:601-5.

Chapter 9: Fever of unknown origin
1. Groopman. How doctors think. A Mariner Book. Houghton Mifflin Company. Boston, 2008.
2. DeAngeles B. What women want men to know. Hyperion, NY 2001.
3. Arush, Rabbi Shalom. Garden of peace. Thread of Mercy Institute, (Hebrew), Jerusalem, Israel, 2008.
4. Sifra Beraita de Rabbi Ishmael Parasha A. (Hebrew) Thirteen rules.
5. Hendrix H: Getting the love you want. An Owl book, Henry Holt and company, NY 1988.
6. Hendrix H: Giving the love that heals. Pocket Books, a division of Simon & Schuster, 1997.
7. Oliver Sacks: Migraine. Picador, UK 1995.
8. Gelfand JA, Callahan MV. Fever of unknown origin. In: Longo DL, Fauci AS, Kaspar DL, Hauser SL, Jameson JL, Loscalzo J, eds. Harrison's Principles and Practice of Internal Medicine. 18st edition. McGraw Hill NY 2012; 158-164.

9. Langford CA, Fauci AS. The vasculitis syndromes. In: Longo DL, Fauci AS, Kaspar DL, Hauser SL, Jameson JL, Loscalzo J, eds. Harrison's Principles and Practice of Internal Medicine. 18st edition. McGraw Hill NY 2012; 2785-2801.
10. Mackowiak PA, Durack DT. Fever of unknown origin. In: Mandell GL, Bennett JE, Dolin R, eds. Mandell, Douglas and Bennett's Principles and Practice of Infectious Diseases. 7th edition. Churchill Livingstone Elsevier, Philadelphia 2010: 779-789.
11. GIDEON expert computer program. http://www.gideononline.com/
12. Bottieau E, Moreira J, Clerinx J, Colebunders R, Van Gompel A, Van den Ende J. Evaluation of the GIDEON expert computer program for the diagnosis of imported febrile illnesses. Med Decis Making. 2008;28:435-42.
13. Duff P, Barth WH Jr, Post MD. Case records of the Massachusetts General Hospital. Case 4-2009. A 39-year-old pregnant woman with fever after a trip to Africa. N Engl J Med. 2009 29;360:508-16.
14. Speil C, Mushtaq A, Adamski A, Khardori N. Fever of unknown origin in the returning traveler. Infect Dis Clin North Am. 2007;21:1091-113.
15. Schmidt WA, Kraft HE, Vorpahl K, Völker L, Gromnica-Ihle EJ. Color duplex ultrasonography in the diagnosis of temporal arteritis. N Engl J Med. 1997; 337:1336-42.

Chapter 10: Leprosy: drug toxicity only?

1. Gelber RH. Leprosy. In: Longo DL, Fauci AS, Kaspar DL, Hauser SL, Jameson JL, Loscalzo J, eds. Harrison's Principles and Practice of Internal Medicine. 18st edition. McGraw Hill NY 2012; 1359-1367.
2. Renault CA, Ernst JD. Mycobacterium leprae. In: Mandell GL, Bennett JE, Dolin R, eds. Mandell, Douglas and Bennett's Principles and Practice of Infectious Diseases. 7th edition. Churchill Livingstone Elsevier, Philadelphia 2010: 3165-76.
3. Yalom ID: Lying on the couch. Harper Perennial. NY 1996.
4. Yalom ID: When Nietzsche wept. Harper Perennial. NY 1992.
5. Yalom ID: Love's executioner. Penguin books UK, 1989.
6. Oscar Wilde: The picture of Dorian Gray. A Modern Library paperback.
7. Maugham WS: The razor's edge. Penguin books, 1972.
8. Grossman Rabbi Z. On the weekly portion (Hebrew). Sifriaty (Gitler) Ltd, Bne Barak, Israel, 1997.
9. Leviticus Chapters 12-14. Leprosy
10. Finkelman Rabbi S, Berkovitz Rabbi I. Chafetz Chaim: The daily lesson. A. Blum Books Ltd, Jerusalem. (Hebrew).
11. Conrad J. Heart of darkness. Dover Publications.
12. Scientific American: Cities. September 2011.
13. Lise Bourbeau: Heal your wounds and find your true self. Editions E.T.C. Inc. Canada.
14. Lise Bourbeau. Listen to your body, your best friend on earth. Editions E.T.C. Inc. Canada 1989.
15. Nsagha DS, Bamgboye EA, Assob JC, et al. Elimination of Leprosy as a public health problem by 2000 AD: an epidemiological perspective. Pan Afr Med J. 2011;9:4.
16. Dacso MM, Jacobson RR, Scollard DM, Stryjewska BM, Prestigiacomo JF. Evaluation of multi-drug therapy for leprosy in the United States using daily rifampin. South Med J. 2011;104:689-94.
17. Setia MS, Shinde SS, Jerajani HR, Boivin JF. Is there a role for rifampicin, ofloxacin and minocycline therapy in the treatment of leprosy? Systematic review and meta-analysis. Trop Med Int Health. 2011 Sep 13.
18. Harris K. Pride and prejudice-identity and stigma in leprosy work. Lepr Rev. 2011;82:135-46.

19. Singh N, Arora VK, Jain A, Bhattacharya SN, Bhatia A. Cytology of testicular changes in leprosy. Acta Cytol. 2002;46:659-63.
20. Gupta SC, Bajaj AK, Singh PA. Testicular biopsy in antispermatozoal antibody positive tuberculoid leprosy patients. Int J Lepr Other Mycobact Dis. 1984;52:255.
21. Yew WW, Leung CC. Antituberculosis drugs and hepatotoxicity. Respirology. 2006;11(6):699-707.
22. de Rosnay P, Irvine LM. Reporting rates of ectopic pregnancy: Are we any closer to achieving consensus? J Obstet Gynaecol. 2012;32:64-7.
23. Fernandes GL, Torloni MR, Hisaba WJ, et al. Premature rupture of membranes before 28 weeks managed expectantly: Maternal and perinatal outcomes in a developing country. J Obstet Gynaecol. 2012;32:45-9.
24. Hernandez AR, Silva CH, Agranonik M, Quadros FM, Goldani MZ. Analysis of infant mortality trends and risk factors in Porto Alegre, Rio Grande do Sul State, Brazil, 1996-2008. Cad Saude Publica. 2011;27:2188-96.

Chapter 11: Second generation syndrome

1. Brom D. The consequences of the Holocaust on child survivors and children of survivors. Isr J Psychiatry Relat Sci. 2001;38:1-2.
2. Brom D, Kfir R, Dasberg H. A controlled double-blind study on children of Holocaust survivors. Isr J Psychiatry Relat Sci. 2001;38:3-12.
3. Cohen M, Brom D, Dasberg H.Child survivors of the Holocaust: symptoms and coping after fifty years. Special section on the consequences of the Holocaust on child survivors and children of survivors. Gefen Pub. House Ltd., 2001.
4. Gordon N. The Physician. Fawcett Crest, NY 1986.
5. Arendt H. Eichmann in Jerusalem: A Report on the Banality of Evil. Penguin Classics.
6. Genesis 37: 1-36. Joseph's sale.
7. Mann T. Joseph and his brothers. Everyman's Library, Alfred A. Knopf, 2005.
8. Abulafia M. On the verge of Eden (Hebrew). Machon Meir, Jerusalem, Israel.
9. Deuteronomy 8:17. Taking pride of prowess.
10. Babylonian Talmud, Additions to Tractate Menachot 30: 2 (Hebrew).
11. Exodus 22: 22-23. Wrongdoing of strangers, widows or orphans.
12. Lewis B. What went wrong? Western impact and Middle-Eastern response.
13. Lewis B. Semites and Anti-Semites: An Inquiry into Conflict and Prejudice.
14. Leviticus 26: 14-46 and Deuteronomy 28: 15-69. Curses.
15. Schwartz-Bart A. The last of the just. Vintage 2001.

Chapter 12: Chronic fatigue syndrome: A case for complimentary medicine

1. Halevy J. Complementary and alternative medicine. All the facts. (Hebrew) Kinneret, Zmora-Bitan, Dvir – Publishing House, Ltd.2005.
2. Singh S and Ernst E. Trick or treatment. The undeniable facts about alternative medicine. Bantam Press, UK, 2008.
3. Servan-Schreiber D. The instinct to heal. Rodale Inc., US 2004.
4. Browning T. The power of softness. Holistic pulsing. Inanna, Australia 2004.
5. Levy M, Editor. I guarantee him. Healing and disease prevention according to the Kingston Clinic (Hebrew). Jerusalem, 2008.
6. Bays B. The Journey. HarperElement, HarperCollinsPublishers Ltd 2003.
7. Siegel BS. Love, medicine and miracles. Arrow Books Limited. Random House, UK 1988.

8. Redfield J: The celestine prophecy. Bantam Books, London UK, 1994.
9. Jenson J: Reclaiming your life. Penguin, USA 1995.
10. Chopra D: Journey into healing. Harmony books, NY 1994.
11. Chopra D: Quantum healing. Exploring the frontiers of mind/body medicine. Bantam books. NY 1990.
12. Peck MS: The road less traveled. Arrow books, 2006.
13. Lievegoed B: Phases: The spiritual rhythms in adult life. Sophia Books, Rudolph Steiner press, 2003.
14. Dawes B, Downing D. Why M.E.? A guide to combating post-viral illness. Grafton Books. London, UK, 1989.
15. Servan-Schreiber D. Anti Cancer. A new way of life. Penguin Books, UK 2007.
16. Weeks N. The medical discoveries of Edward Bach, physician. C.W. Daniel Company Ltd. UK, 1973.
17. Epstein Rosen L, Amador XF. When someone you love is depressed. How to help your loved one without losing yourself. A Fireside trade paperback. Simon & Schuster. NY, 1996.
18. Hahnemann S: Organon of medicine. B. Jain Publishers (PVT), Ltd. New Delhi, India 1997.
19. Kent JT. Repertory of the homoeopathic material medica and a word index. Jain Publishers (PVT), Ltd. New Delhi, India 1996.
20. Sankaran R. The soul of remedies. Homoeopathic Medical Publishers, Mumbai, India 2004.
21. Sankaran R. The sensation in homoeopathy. Homoeopathic Medical Publishers, Mumbai, India 2005.
22. Engleberg NC. Chronic fatigue syndrome. In: Mandell GL, Bennett JE, Dolin R, eds. Mandell, Douglas and Bennett's Principles and Practice of Infectious Diseases. 7th edition. Churchill Livingstone Elsevier, Philadelphia 2010: 1877-1904.
23. Constant EL, Adam S, Gillain B, Lambert M, Masquelier E, Seron X. Cognitive deficits in patients with chronic fatigue syndrome compared to those with major depressive disorder and healthy controls. Clin Neurol Neurosurg. 2011;113:295-302.
24. Landier W, Tse AM. Use of complementary and alternative medical interventions for the management of procedure-related pain, anxiety, and distress in pediatric oncology: an integrative review. J Pediatr Nurs. 2010;25:566-79.
25. Fukuda K, Nisenbaum R, Stewart G, et al. Chronic multisymptom illness affecting Air Force veterans of the Gulf War. JAMA. 1998;280:981-8.
26. Jones JF, Maloney EM, Boneva RS, Jones AB, Reeves WC. Complementary and alternative medical therapy utilization by people with chronic fatiguing illnesses in the United States. BMC Complement Altern Med. 2007;7:12.
27. Mease P. Fibromyalgia syndrome: review of clinical presentation, pathogenesis, outcome measures, and treatment. J Rheumatol Suppl. 2005;75:6-21.
28. Briere J, Jordan CE. Childhood maltreatment, intervening variables, and adult psychological difficulties in women: an overview. Trauma Violence Abuse. 2009;10:375-88.

Chapter 13: Chronic urinary tract infection: What if ovaries could speak?
1. Bays B: The Journey. Harper Element, London 1999.
2. Browning T. Femophobia. How women have become men. Innana, 2005.
3. Kunin CM. Urinary-catheter-associated infections in the elderly. Int J Antimicrob Agents. 2006;28 Suppl 1:S78-81.
4. Gupta K, Trautner BW. Urinary tract infection, pyelonephritis and prostatitis. In: Longo DL, Fauci AS, Kaspar DL, Hauser SL, Jameson JL, Loscalzo J, eds. Harrison's Principles and Practice of Internal Medicine. 18st edition. McGraw Hill NY 2012; 2387-2395.

5. Sobel J, Kaye D. Urinary tract infections. In: Mandell GL, Bennett JE, Dolin R, eds. Mandell, Douglas and Bennett's Principles and Practice of Infectious Diseases. 7th edition. Churchill Livingstone Elsevier, Philadelphia 2010: 957-85.
6. Bahagon Y, Raveh D, Schlesinger Y, Rudensky B, Yinnon AM. Bacteremic urinary tract infection in emergency department patients: Prevalence and predictive features. Eur J Clin Microbiol Infect Dis 2007; 26: 349-352.
7. Raveh D, Yinnon AM, Broide E, Rudensky B. Susceptibilities of ESBL-producing Enterobacteriaceae to Ertapenem, meropenem, and piperacillin-tazobactam, with and without clavulanic acid. Chemotherapy 2007; 53: 185-189.
8. Cohen MJ, Anshilevitz O, Raveh D, Broide E, Rudensky B, Yinnon AM. Colonization and acquisition of multi-drug resistant organisms among hospital patients neighboring the critically ill. Infect Contr Hosp Epidemiol 2006; 27: 675-681.
9. Raveh D, Rosenzweig I, Rudensky B, Yinnon AM. Prospective, case control study to determine risk factors for community-acquired urinary tract infection due to *Pseudomonas aeruginosa* or *Enterococcus*. Eur J Clin Microbiol Infect Dis 2006; 25: 331-334.
10. Henschke R, Yinnon AM, Rudensky B, Attias D, Raveh D. Assessment of the clinical significance of production of Extended-Spectrum-β-lactamase (ESBL) by Enterobacteriaceae. Infection 2006; 34: 66-74.
11. Benenson S, Yinnon AM, Schlesinger Y, Rudensky B, Raveh D. Optimization of empirical antibiotic selection for suspected Gram-negative bacteremia in the emergency department. Int J Antimicrobiol Ag 2005; 25:398-403.

Chapter 14: Peyronie's disease: Transforming weakness to strength
1. Schwartz-Bart A, The last of the Just. Vintage classics.
2. Leviticus 26: 14-46 and Deuteronomy 28: 15-69.
3. Axline VM. Dibs, in search of self.
4. Miller A. The Drama of the Gifted Child: The Search for the True Self.
5. Bible. Hosea Chapter 1-3. Hosea's tragedy.
6. Steinsaltz A. The thirteen petalled rose. A discourse on the essence of Jewish existence and belief. Basic Books, Inc 2006.
7. Yalkut Shimoni, Yeshayahu 246:490 (Hebrew).
8. Dibenedetti DB, Nguyen D, Zografos L, Ziemiecki R, Zhou X. A Population-Based Study of Peyronie's Disease: Prevalence and Treatment Patterns in the United States. Adv Urol. 2011;2011:282503. Epub 2011 Oct 23.
9. Kuehhas FE, Weibl P, Georgi T, Djakovic N, Herwig R. Peyronie's Disease: Non-surgical Therapy Options. Rev Urol. 2011;13:139-46.
10. Abern MR, Larsen S, Levine LA. Combination of Penile Traction, Intralesional Verapamil, and Oral Therapies for Peyronie's Disease. J Sex Med. 2011 Oct 24.
11. Paulis G, D'Ascenzo R, Nupieri P, et al. Effectiveness of antioxidants (propolis, blueberry, vitamin E) associated with verapamil in the medical management of Peyronie's disease: a study of 151 cases. Int J Androl. 2011 Sep 27.
12. Serefoglu EC, Hellstrom WJ. Treatment of Peyronie's disease: 2012 update. Curr Urol Rep. 2011;12:444-52.
13. Larsen SM, Levine LA. Peyronie's disease: review of nonsurgical treatment options. Urol Clin North Am. 2011;38:195-205.

14. LeRoy TJ, Broderick GA. Doppler blood flow analysis of erectile function: who, when, and how. Urol Clin North Am. 2011;38:147-54.
15. Barnhill A. What it takes to defend deceptive placebo use. Kennedy Inst Ethics J. 2011;21:219-50.
16. Zhang HL. Placebo - More hatred than love. J Neurosci Rural Pract. 2011;2:105-7.
17. Kupferschmidt K. More placebo use promoted in Germany. CMAJ. 2011 12; 183:E633-4.
18. Kirsch I. The use of placebos in clinical trials and clinical practice. Can J Psychiatry. 2011;56:191-2.
19. Roustit C, Campoy E, Renahy E, King G, Parizot I, Chauvin P. Family social environment in childhood and self-rated health in young adulthood. BMC Public Health. 2011 22;11:949.

Chapter 15: A case of marital conflict and distress
1. Gray J. Men are from Mars, women are from Venus. Harper Collins Publishers, 1995.
2. Davidovitch D. The Ketuba. Jewish marriage contracts through the ages. E. Lewin-Epstein Ltd, Publishers, Tel Aviv, Israel 1979.
3. The exact prayer book (Siddur), 4th edition. Machon HaRav Mazliach. Bne Barak, Israel. 2006: 216-218 (Hebrew). Ramban's letter to his son.
4. Sayings of the Fathers (Mishnah/Pirkeh Avoth): chapter 4: 1. Honorable man
5. Rashi, Exodus: 20:21.
6. Ginzburgh Rabbi I. The marriage contract (Hebrew). Gal Einai Institute, Israel.
7. McCullough JP Jr, Lord BD, Martin AM, Conley KA, Schramm E, Klein DN. The significant other history: an interpersonal-emotional history procedure used with the early-onset chronically depressed patient. Am J Psychother. 2011;65:225-48.
8. Rees CA. All they need is love? Helping children to recover from neglect and abuse. Arch Dis Child. 2011;96:969-76.
9. Rees CA. Understanding emotional abuse. Arch Dis Child. 2010;95:59-67.
10. Gostecnik C, Repic T. Relational marital paradigm. Am J Psychother. 2009;63:1-12.
11. Hills L. Defusing the angry patient: 25 tips. J Med Pract Manage. 2010;26:158-62
12. Mienaltowski A, Corballis PM, Blanchard-Fields F, Parks NA, Hilimire MR. Anger management: age differences in emotional modulation of visual processing. Psychol Aging. 2011;26:224-31.

Chapter 16: Suicide: A story of jealousy and ambition
1. Arush Rabbi S: Garden of Peace. (Hebrew) Thread of Mercy Institute, Jerusalem, Israel 2008.
2. Arush Rabbi S: The wisdom of women. (Hebrew) Thread of Mercy Institute, Jerusalem, Israel 2009.
3. Davidovitch D. The Ketuba. Jewish marriage contracts through the ages. E. Lewin-Epstein Ltd, Publishers, Tel Aviv, Israel 1979.
4. Malca H. Towards Shabath. An internal view into the weekly Torah portion. (Hebrew) Beer Shevah, Israel. 2006
5. The essential Rabbi Nahman. Breslev.co.il.
6. Genesis: Genesis 29: 17 and 31-24 and 35:16-20. Rachel and Lea.
7. Genesis 4: 2-16. Cain and Abel
8. Genesis: 3: 16. Passion for your husband.
9. Genesis: 2: 18. A helper against himself.
10. Genesis 37: 5-11. Joseph's dreams
11. Genesis 17: 1. Walking innocent before God
12. Genesis 24: 67. Isaac loves Rivka, is consoled after Sarah's death.
13. Genesis 29: 22-35 and 30: 1-24 and 35: 16-19. Jacob with Laban and marriage with his two wives,

14. Freud, superego
15. Sayings of the Fathers (Mishnah/Pirkeh Avoth): chapter 4: 21. Jealousy, passion and honor.
16. Sayings of the Fathers (Mishnah/Pirkeh Avoth): chapter 4: 21. Conquering one's instincts.
17. Genesis 22:1. Abraham's tribulations
18. Smith JC, Curry SC. Prolonged toxicity after amitriptyline overdose in a patient deficient in CYP2D6 activity. J Med Toxicol. 2011;7:220-3.
19. Güloglu C, Orak M, Ustündag M, Altunci YA. Analysis of amitriptyline overdose in emergency medicine. Emerg Med J. 2011;28:296-9.
20. Stübner S, Grohmann R, von Stralendorff I, et al. Suicidality as rare adverse event of antidepressant medication: report from the AMSP multicenter drug safety surveillance project. J Clin Psychiatry. 2010;71:1293-307.
21. Hawton K, Bergen H, Simkin S, et al. Toxicity of antidepressants: rates of suicide relative to prescribing and non-fatal overdose. Br J Psychiatry. 2010;196:354-8.
22. Simkin S, Hawton K, Kapur N, Gunnell D. What can be done to reduce mortality from paracetamol overdoses? A patient interview study. QJM. 2012;105:41-51.
23. Hawton K, Bergen H, Simkin S, et al. Impact of different pack sizes of paracetamol in the United Kingdom and Ireland on intentional overdoses: a comparative study. BMC Public Health. 2011;11:460.
24. Manthripragada AD, Zhou EH, Budnitz DS, Lovegrove MC, Willy ME. Characterization of acetaminophen overdose-related emergency department visits and hospitalizations in the United States. Pharmacoepidemiol Drug Saf. 2011;20:819-26.
25. Altarescu G, Barenholz O, Renbaum P, et al. Preimplantation genetic diagnosis (PGD)--prevention of the birth of children affected with endocrine diseases. J Pediatr Endocrinol Metab. 2011;24:543-8.
26. Altarescu G, Reish O, Renbaum P, et al. Preimplantation genetic diagnosis (PGD) for SHOX-related haploinsufficiency in conjunction with trisomy 21 detection by molecular analysis. J Assist Reprod Genet. 2011;28:233-8.

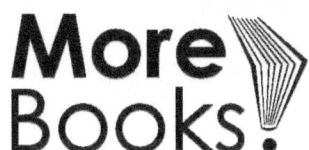
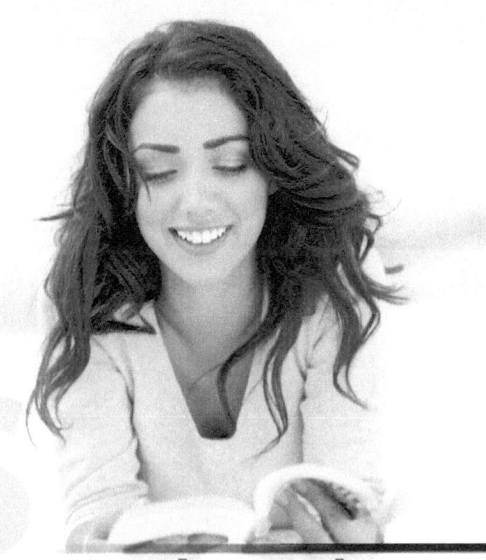

I want morebooks!

Buy your books fast and straightforward online - at one of the world's fastest growing online book stores! Environmentally sound due to Print-on-Demand technologies.

Buy your books online at

www.get-morebooks.com

Kaufen Sie Ihre Bücher schnell und unkompliziert online – auf einer der am schnellsten wachsenden Buchhandelsplattformen weltweit!
Dank Print-On-Demand umwelt- und ressourcenschonend produziert.

Bücher schneller online kaufen

www.morebooks.de

OmniScriptum Marketing DEU GmbH
Heinrich-Böcking-Str. 6-8
D - 66121 Saarbrücken
Telefax: +49 681 93 81 567-9

info@omniscriptum.com
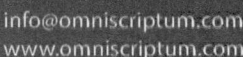
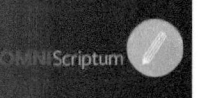

www.ingramcontent.com/pod-product-compliance
Lightning Source LLC
Chambersburg PA
CBHW020653220526
45464CB00001B/416